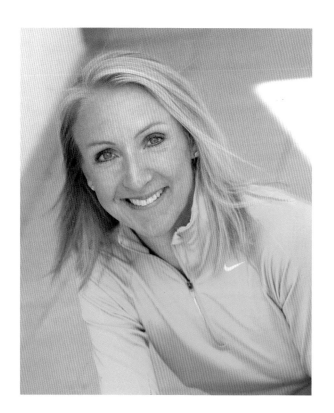

HOW TO RUN

SIMON &
SCHUSTER
ILLUSTRATED

London · New York · Sydney · Toronto

A CBS COMPANY

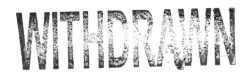

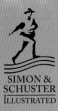

SIMON & SCHUSTER
ILLUSTRATED

First published in Great Britain by Simon & Schuster UK Ltd, 2011
A CBS COMPANY

1 3 5 7 9 10 8 6 4 2

SIMON & SCHUSTER
ILLUSTRATED BOOKS
Simon & Schuster UK Ltd
222 Gray's Inn Road
London WC1X 8HB

www.simonandschuster.co.uk

Simon & Schuster Australia
Sydney

A CIP catalogue record for this book is available from the British Library

ISBN 978-1-84737-074-7

Editorial director: Francine Lawrence
Project editor: Hilary Ivory
Design: XAB Design
Production manager: Katherine Thornton

Photo credits

Photographs by Ruth Jenkinson except for:
Victah Sailer, Photo Run: pp. 4, 6–7, 83, 109, 118–19, 123, 124–5, 126–7
bilderlounge/Alessandro Ventura/Getty Images: p. 76
Monalyn Gracia/Corbis: p. 172

Printed and bound in U.A.E.

DISCLAIMER

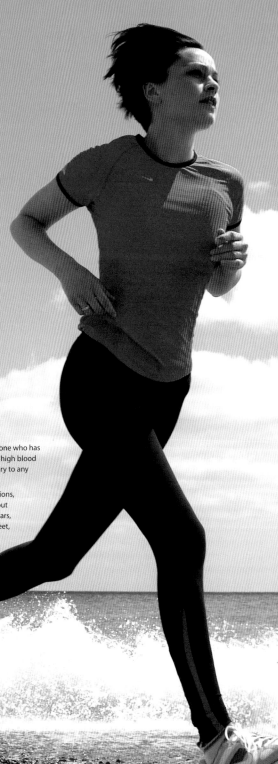

how to run

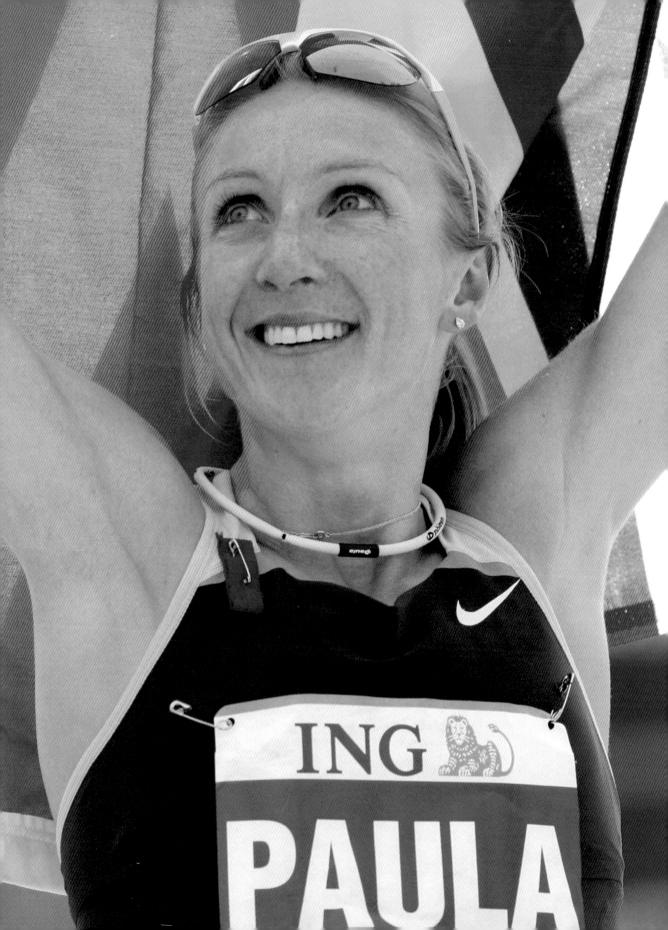

introduction

One of the first things people ask me is why I run. It's actually a difficult question to answer – not because I don't know why, but because there are so many reasons that it's difficult to get them all across in words.

To me, running is not just something that I do – it is a huge part of my life, of who I am. It is my passion, my stress relief, one of my greatest loves. It makes me feel better about myself and gives me a more positive outlook on life. It keeps me healthy and strong and makes me feel a more balanced person. Yes, it has brought me a lot of success, but by far the most important factor is the amount of fun and enjoyment it has given me.

It's for all these reasons that I want to share my love of running with you and help you get the most out of your own efforts.

Let's face it: running is one of the simplest and easiest sports to take up. It's also one of the most effective forms of exercise. You need very little equipment and can do it almost anywhere, any time. It's one of the best ways to stay fit and healthy. There's no time wasted getting to and from gyms – you do it where you want, according to your own timetable, at your pace. Yet it's more than that: I think of running as *my time* – time for me to relax and enjoy, when I do some of my best thinking. I feel more free and alive than at any other time because of the increased oxygen pumping around my body. My senses are awake and alert; I appreciate the surroundings better, notice colours more vibrantly and often solve problems, conundrums or dilemmas that initially seemed insurmountable and were driving me crazy indoors.

Another question people ask is when did I first begin running. Again, this is a tough one to answer. It's easier to say that I don't remember a time when I didn't run. Almost as soon as I could walk I discovered that it was a lot more fun to run. At school sports days it was always the running events that I loved and, from a very early age, I remember the magical feeling of running fast through forests. No surprise, then, that the first sports club I wanted to join was the athletics club. I still remember my first proper race – a cross-country event – the buzz and the way it made me feel. I didn't win that one, but that didn't matter one bit. What did matter was the way it made me feel so invigorated and alive. I loved the sensation of running hard, the idea of challenging my body, mind and spirit to work in harmony and carry me over the ground as fast as possible.

Of course there are many reasons why people run, and everyone will have their own particular motivation that drives them out there. However, what really keeps so many people running is that once they have discovered the sheer joy of it, they are quite simply hooked. In return, running keeps you fit, toned and healthy, brings you a longer life expectancy and a whole new circle of friends. In short, it helps make you a more confident and positive person.

You may be thinking about starting running simply to get healthier or to lose weight. You may want to take up something that will give you valuable 'me time' and make you feel better about yourself. You may already be a runner, but thinking about taking the next step and trying a race. Or you may be an established racer looking for ideas on improving your times. Whatever your level or goal, I hope there will be something in this book to help you. That, for me, is one of the most beautiful things about running – it unites so many people and ability levels in one simple action. In what other sport can you have over 35,000 people taking part in the same race, at the same place, and at the same time, all going through similar emotions, trials and experiences? That's why nothing beats the feeling of empathy and understanding, the atmosphere of camaraderie and sharing, and the achievement that we feel at the end of a race.

Paula Radcliffe

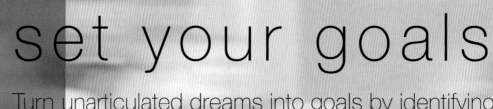

1 set your goals

Turn unarticulated dreams into goals by identifying why you want them. Nothing ignites your ambitions more forcefully than when you consciously give them shape and form.

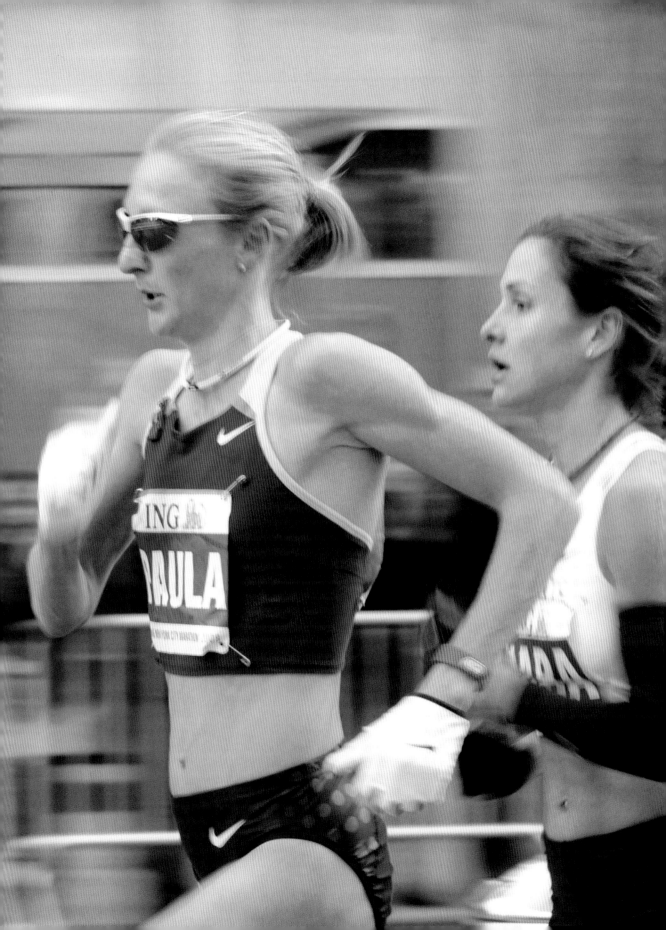

set your goals

Before I begin laying out the basics of how to get started, you first need to look within yourself and think about your own personal aims and goals: what do you want to get out of your running?

Like anything in life, you're far more likely to derive satisfaction and enjoyment from whatever you're doing and, also, get the most from yourself, if you have a definite reason or motive to keep going.

When I was a teenager I got into the habit every New Year of writing down my goals for the year ahead on a piece of paper that I'd fold and keep in my yearly training diary. Some were running related; others were to do with my personal or school life. From time to time I'd look at the list to see how I was doing and then, at the end of the year, I'd get it out and review how many of my aims I had achieved. I don't think I ever achieved all of them, but that's not a bad thing: had I achieved them all, I'd have felt that I hadn't been aiming high enough or stretching myself hard enough.

'The best way to get started is to stop talking and begin doing'

Walt Disney

I had two sections to the list: realistic goals and dream goals. Dream goals were achievements I really desired, but that were always going to be very, very hard for me. But I understood that if I didn't at least have a go at achieving them, I'd have no chance at all of turning dreams into reality. It's a fact that if we don't stretch ourselves we'll never know what we're really capable of. One of my favourite sayings is: 'Aim for the moon, because even if you miss, you'll land among the stars'. It doesn't matter if you don't attain the highest dream goal – you'll always achieve more on the journey than you'd ever have done by aiming only for what you know you can pull off. Besides, you'll discover a host of other valuable insights into yourself and others along the way. Our bodies are designed to react to stress by upping the ante and becoming more efficient and effective. By identifying what really lights a fire within you, you are acknowledging the existence of something that you very much want. This will make it more likely that you'll be happy to put in the work and push yourself hard to try and achieve it.

Your aim may simply be to get fitter, lose weight or improve your general health. It may be to run a mile or to finish a marathon; run a certain distance faster than you have ever run it before; or just get out of the house and have half an hour to yourself a few times a week without the intrusion of work or family hassles. Whatever it is, I guarantee that you'll get more out of your running if, right from the beginning, you have established a reason for why you're doing it and what you want to get out of it.

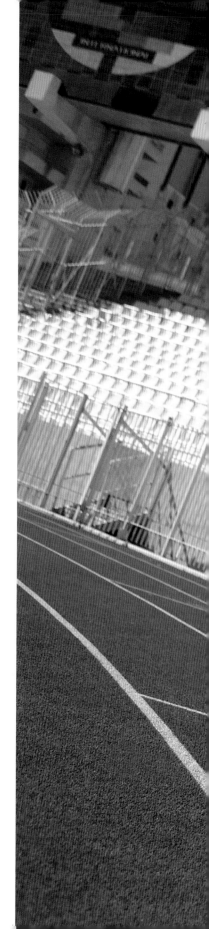

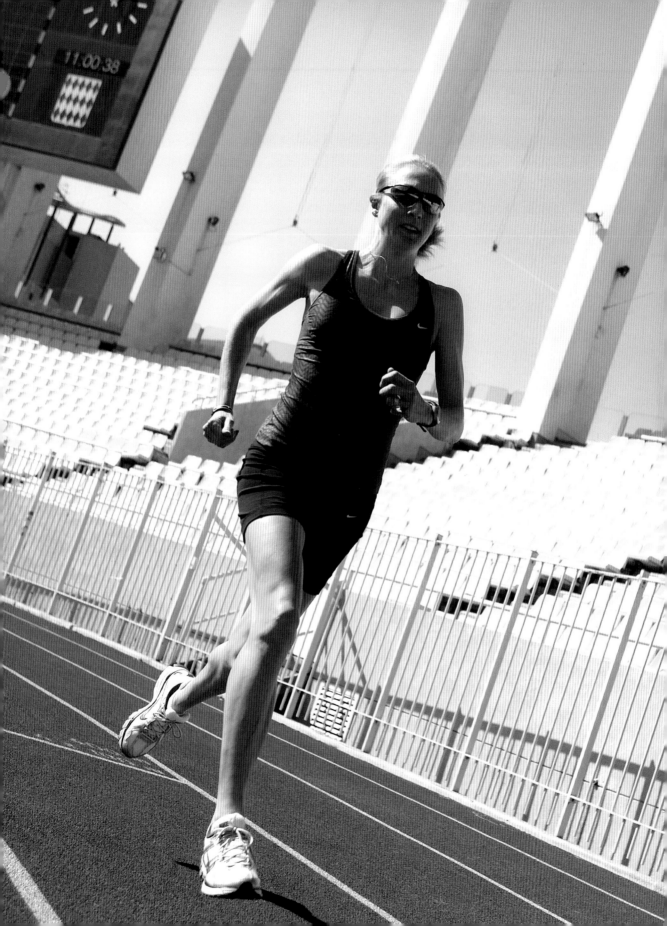

Step 1 **Set out your ultimate goal/s**

Write the big ones down in longhand rather than typing them on to a computer screen. Longhand slows down your thought processes, giving the brain time to focus on one thing and setting it apart from the clutter that overwhelms the mind the rest of the time. This way, your brain has a chance to analyse what you are writing and make decisions while you're doing it. It allows you greater control over your thought processes and provides your brain with an image to visualise during the really tough times. Use positive words to express your goals: for example, rather than negative commands such as 'Stop smoking', turn the phrasing around and it becomes 'Clean up my lungs'. By re-orienting your mindset, you focus on the happy outcome rather than the prevailing situation.

Step 2 **Visualise your goals**

What is it about this goal that will make such a difference to your life? Picture yourself after you've achieved it… How will you feel? What will people say?

Most of us tend to be mentally focused on how things are now, repeating the same thoughts to ourselves throughout the course of our lives. What this does is perpetuate the same set of circumstances, preserving our version of 'reality'. I've heard psychologists comparing this with watching the same film over and over again. But we're not locked into this pattern: we have the tools to change it right within our grasp, the most effective of which is the imagination. All we have to do is unleash its power and set about visualising circumstances that are different. This way, we change what we think of as our day-to-day 'reality'; in the process, we discover that it's just one version of many different 'realities'.

The unconscious mind doesn't distinguish between a real experience and a vividly imagined one: running through how the outcome will make us feel will also have the effect of bringing us closer to achieving it.

I use this technique a lot in race preparation. I visualise how I might act in a few scenarios that could unfold during the race (always calmly and in control); and I consistently conjure up a vision of myself crossing the finish line in the best possible shape and form.

Step 3 **Set yourself a few smaller, more easily achieved goals**

Smaller goals act as stepping-stones along the way to achieving the bigger one, and picking them off one by one will have an extraordinarily positive effect on the pursuit of your primary objective. Setting a goal that's too high – for example, running a marathon in eight weeks' time when you haven't put in the groundwork – is doomed to failure and/or injury, not to mention demoralisation. We are impatient creatures by and large, and we tend to expect success the minute we put our trainers on. But the old adage of avoiding doing 'too much, too soon, too quickly' is one that's best learned sooner, rather than later. In my early running career I was very lucky to have a wise coach who firmly believed in making gradual, steady progression: we were always careful to add only small amounts to the training schedule each year, and to leave room for me to add on more in the future.

With these stepping-stone goals in place, you'll receive a confidence boost every time you achieve one of them. This will give you a physical and mental push towards the next goal.

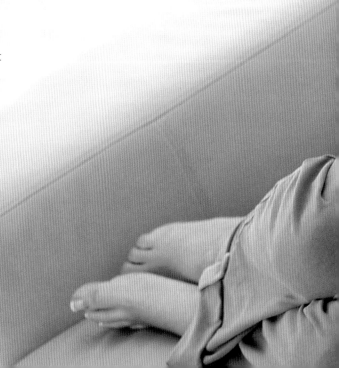

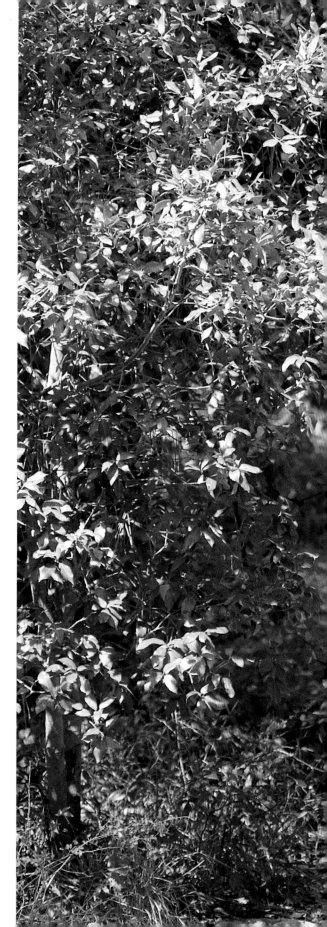

Step 4 Plan how you're going to fit training into your day

Everyone is madly busy, so putting together an action plan is a practical necessity. Schedule fixed time in your weekly diary to pursue your goal, exactly as you would make a note of meetings, lunches or dental appointments; otherwise before you know it the day is over and you won't have made it out of the door. Think about what down-time you have – you may be lucky enough to work in an office with a shower, for instance, in which case you could run to work or run at lunchtime. Keep some spare kit at the office as well as at home, so you have options whenever a window of opportunity crops up. Most importantly, identify the time of day that works best for you. Personally, I prefer to get my best run done in the morning when I feel fresh, enjoying the morning air, setting myself up and feeling good for the day. However, if you are not a morning person, there's no sense in forcing yourself out at the crack of dawn just because that fits neatly with your diary – you'll hate it and will quickly turn against running. Pick the days and times that work best for you and then work them into your week.

'I prefer to get my best run done in the morning when I feel fresh'

Step 5 Re-evaluate and reassess your goals

Without this necessary re-tuning and refinement you risk floundering or floating aimlessly. As you achieve each goal, reward yourself and feel justifiably proud, then get down to setting the next one immediately. If your aims and desires change, then be quick to identify this and modify the goal accordingly. Similarly, if external factors crop up, don't be afraid to alter the goal or timescale. For instance, illness (your own or within your family), injury, and upheaval at work or in your personal life are all going to affect your energy levels, health and vitality. You shouldn't push too hard at these times, nor should you consider giving up your goals totally. Rather, take a step back, modify the goal and reassess the time plan.

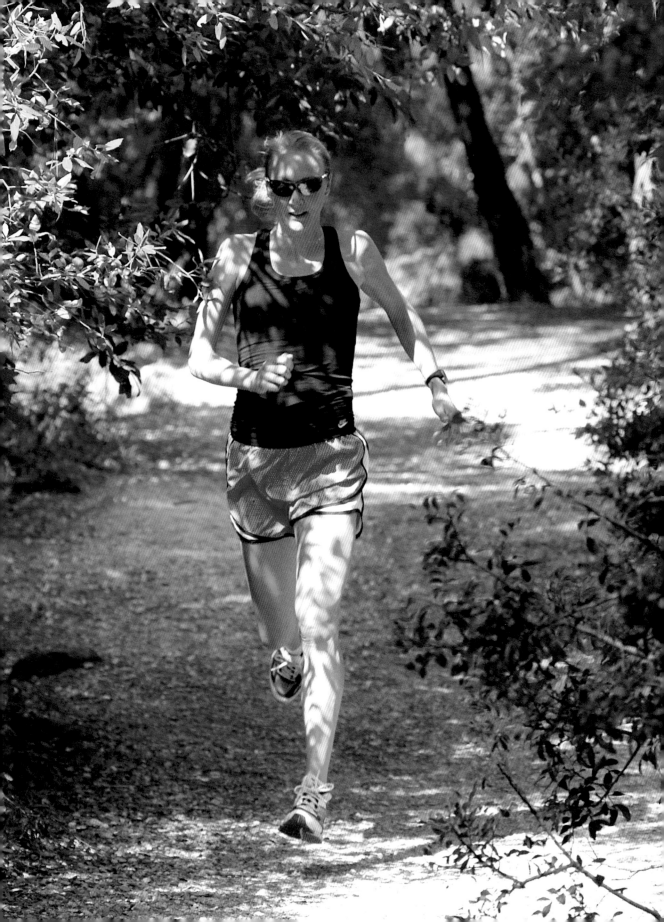

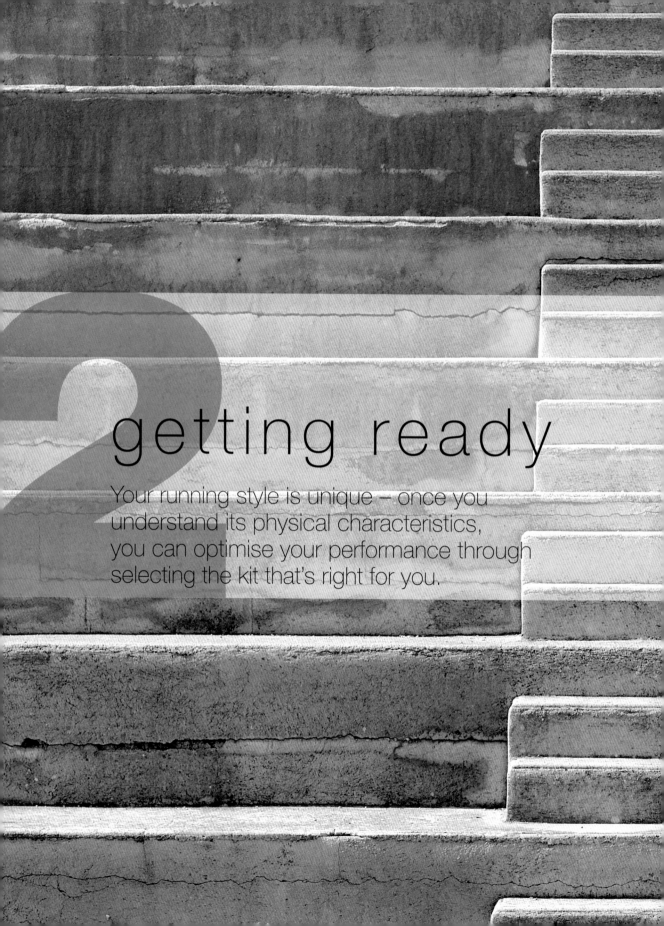

getting ready

Your running style is unique – once you
understand its physical characteristics,
you can optimise your performance through
selecting the kit that's right for you.

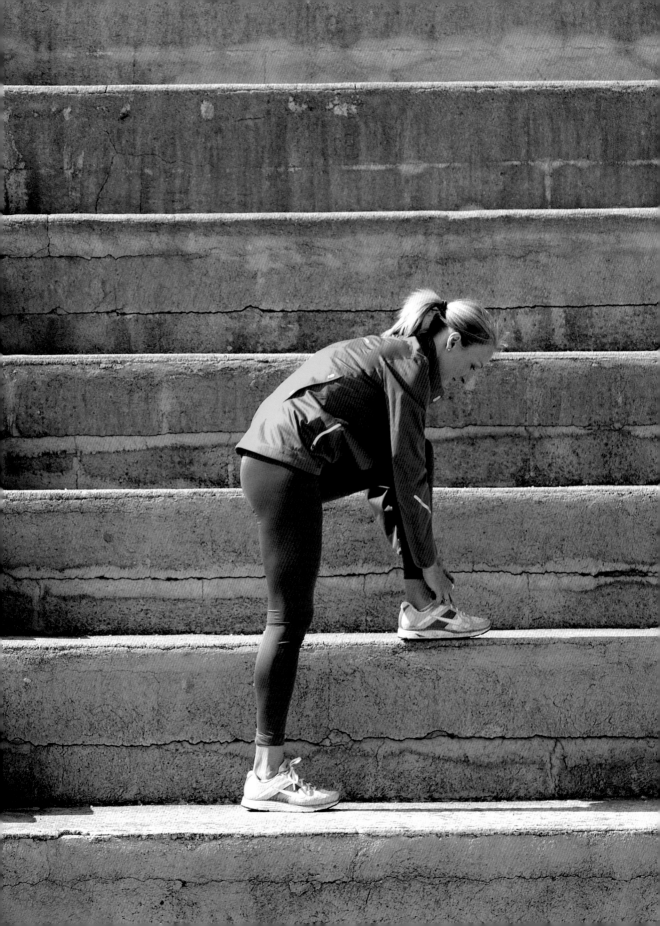

get familiar with your feet

Running is a relatively undemanding sport when you think about how little kit you need, but at the top of the list, and of crucial importance, are the shoes in which you run. Each foot has 26 bones, 33 joints, 107 ligaments and 19 muscles and tendons.

When these components are all working in harmony, your feet will carry you over hill and dale without a great deal of grumbling. But to enable them to perform at their best, they need proper care and attention.

Everyone has a slightly different running style, so it's critically important to choose a shoe that suits the way you, personally, run. Trying to run in tennis or gym shoes – or worse, in fashion trainers – is just asking for injury. Your shoes need to be fit for purpose; this means they should be designed specifically to suit the surface on which you're running, and also the biomechanics of your individual foot-strike pattern.

HOW TO CHOOSE THE RIGHT SHOES

As you'd expect, research and development constantly bring about technological improvements, so the choice of running shoe has expanded exponentially over time. I've been running competitively for over 20 years, so I've had a long time to find out exactly which type of shoe works best for me. Don't be afraid to get an expert's opinion. When you shop for your first pair, go to a specialist running shop where your gait can be observed – this will help you find the particular shoe that's right for you.

Let me pass on what I've learned about selecting the right running shoes.

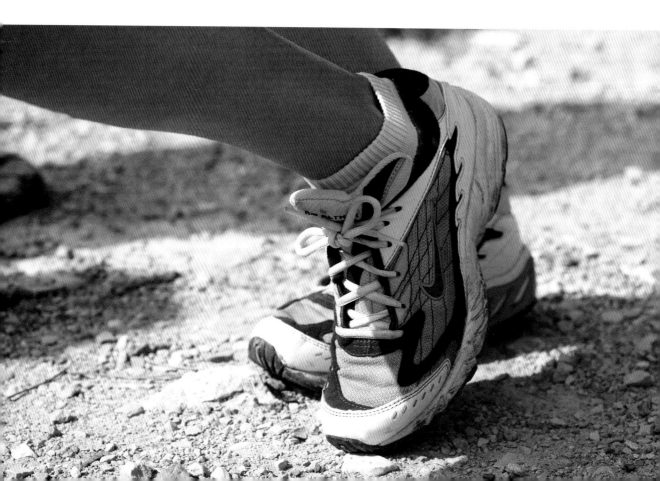

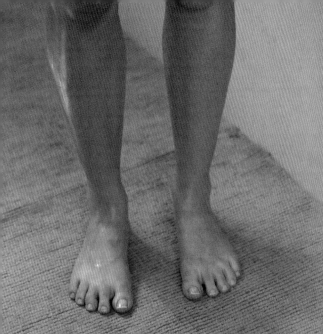

Next time you get out of the shower, plant a wet foot on the bathmat and take a look at the imprint it makes. This will give you a pretty accurate idea of your habitual foot plant and its shape.

If you have high arches you'll see a very narrow imprint under the mid-foot; if you have flat feet you'll see a thick imprint connecting the heel and forefoot; a normal foot will reveal a narrower imprint connecting the heel and forefoot (but not as narrow as a high arch). However, this only describes your foot type; the next step is to analyse your gait – in other words, the way your foot behaves as you land and push off with each stride. How many of us can boast the perfect stride? I wish I could. Check which of these descriptions fits you:

what sort of runner are you?

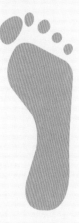 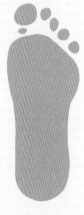 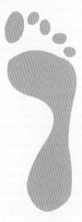

The neutral runner

lands either on their heel or mid-foot, transitions smoothly and efficiently through the arch, then pushes off from the ball of the foot; most of the propulsion force comes from between the first and second toes. The arch flattens a little to absorb their body weight and then springs back, with the foot and ankle staying nicely aligned. Old pairs of shoes will have an even wear pattern.

The overpronator

lands on the outside of the heel and then rolls excessively inwards to the inside of the mid-foot, before pushing off from the inside of the foot. (Over-pronators produce a wet imprint that looks flat-footed.) This running style places a lot of pressure on knees, ankles and hips unless the runner chooses a shoe with an anti-pronation posting (a firmer area that's generally manufactured in a darker colour on the inside of the heel/mid-section of the shoe) plus, possibly, orthotic inserts to support and correct their body alignment as they run. The worn area on their old shoes will typically be on the inside of the soles.

The supinator

lands on the outside of the foot and then either transitions through to toe-off correctly, or rolls in too far and overpronates. (Supinators produce a wet imprint that looks like a high arch, with only the outside edge in contact with the floor.) They need a wider forefoot outsole to prevent them from rolling too much. If they then overpronate, they need a shoe that supports both factors. Some people (I'm one of them) land in supination, but then correct to a neutral style of push-off. Unless they wear shoes with a wide forefoot outsole, they can be prone to turned ankles. As you'd expect, old shoes will show a wear pattern on the outer side of the sole.

what's your foot-strike like?

Within each group there are also heel-strikers and midfoot or forefoot strikers. Heel-strikers hit the ground with their heels and roll through to push-off. Midfoot/forefoot strikers rarely touch the ground with their heels, especially when running fast, and have shorter ground-contact time.

Runners who heel-strike need to pay more attention to the support and cushioning of the heel area.

A good test is to put your old running shoes on a flat, flush surface and look at them at eye level from behind. If they sit evenly, you're a neutral runner; if they tilt inwards, you're an overpronator; if they tilt outwards, you're a supinator.

Runners who have either very broad or very narrow feet should choose from the models that offer wide and narrow options, such as Nike's Pegasus and Structure Triax. If you're particularly heavy or light, there are specially designed running shoes with, accordingly, more or less cushioning.

If you're running shorter distances at faster paces, or you're racing, you might want to consider a shoe that's more responsive and allows you to feel the ground better in order to get greater return on your impact force. This means that more of the energy force with which you strike the ground is returned to your body as you push off, rather than being absorbed by the shoe's cushioning and lost in the ground. (The same reason that running on soft surfaces is slower than on road.) Lastly, if your running gait is extreme and you exaggeratedly overpronate or supinate, consult a biomechanist to see whether orthotic inserts might help stabilise your gait, possibly saving your hips, knees, ankles and lower back from future trouble.

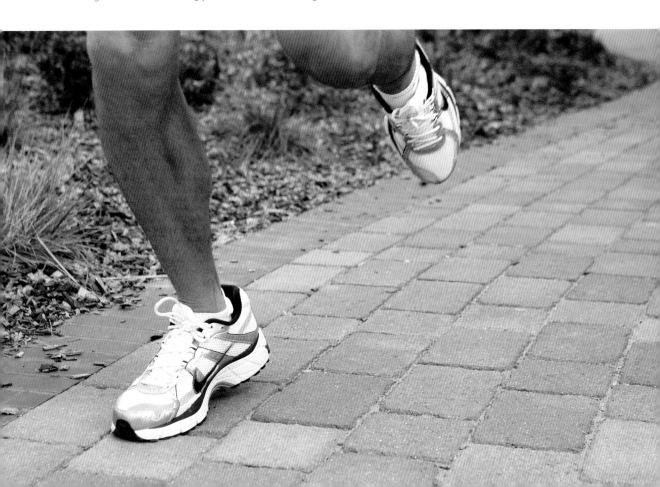

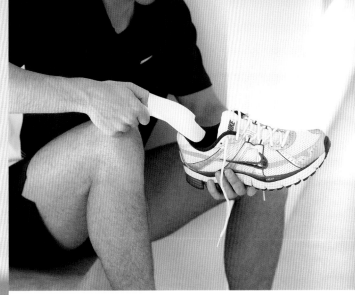

'I'm lucky in that I'm a pretty neutral runner once I have my orthoses in my shoes'

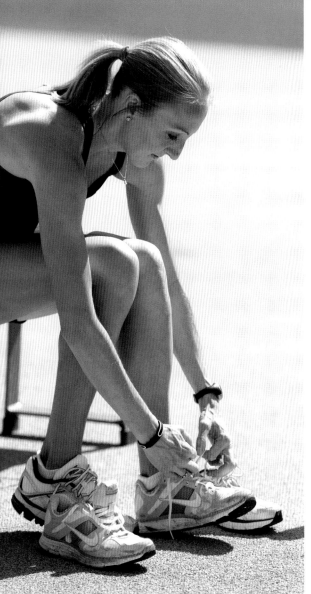

People often ask which shoes I run in. I'm lucky in that I'm a pretty neutral runner once I have my orthoses in my shoes. I'm a forefoot striker and I supinate on both sides, correcting perfectly to toe-off on the right foot and slightly over-correcting to pronate a little on the left foot. My orthoses correct this and give me some arch support. (I had a collapsed arch on the left foot 16 years ago, and to support this I'm rarely without my orthotic inserts.) So, with my orthoses I have a wide choice of shoes. My favourites are the Nike Women's Pegasus and Trail Pegasus, Women's Span, Women's Althea, Nike LunarGlide, Zoom Marathoner, Lunar Elite, Zoom Streak, Zoom Plus and the Free. I like to rotate my shoes, as I find that on different runs I'm looking for different things from them. If I'm tired I want a more cushioned run to protect my legs and help recovery, while if I'm running at a faster pace I look for a lighter, more responsive shoe. If I'm doing fast work or repetitions I go for a racing shoe like the Zoom Marathoner, Streak or Lunar Elite. And if I'm heading off-road where it's likely to be muddy, I'll select a trail shoe.

I also vary my shoes to give my feet a slight change each time. Change is good for your feet, as it stimulates them to get stronger. Your feet and leg muscles will work slightly differently in each different style of shoe, so by changing regularly, you stop your feet becoming lazy or dangerously adapted to one particular shoe. (If the shoe is suddenly discontinued, you're in trouble!)

I am very lucky, because in 2004 I had the chance to work with the Nike shoe designers on the Zoom Marathoner. They were great at incorporating my feedback. As such, it's my perfect racing shoe and it gives me huge confidence to stand on the start line knowing that one thing I never have to worry about is whether I'm wearing the right shoes.

if the shoe fits, wear it

Having the right shoes for your foot type and gait, the terrain on which you run and, importantly, getting them correctly fitted will make the difference between a comfortable and an uncomfortable run.

Crucially, these considerations will also give you either an injury-free or an injury-prone experience. So, let me pass on a few tips that I've found useful.

A good running shop should employ knowledgeable staff who are trained to observe your gait and advise on a selection to suit you. Take an old pair of running shoes with you so that the wear pattern can be scrutinised. The best retailers will ask you to run up and down the shop floor – or treadmill, if they have one – to observe your running style. Never be afraid to ask to try out shoes before you buy; even if you only run up and down on the pavement outside, you'll at least get an idea of whether they fit comfortably. The shoes you choose are the key to getting the most from your running, so take your time and get it right.

If you run mostly on roads or concrete, look for a shoe with more cushioning and a less rugged outsole. However, for running on trails or parkland paths it's better to have a more rugged outsole that will give you more grip, and a shoe that sits a bit closer to the ground to allow you to feel more in control on rougher terrain. Being closer to the ground helps improve your proprioception (i.e. your brain's ability to sense the position, location and orientation of your body). This, in turn, controls your reaction to bumps and dips on the running surface, enabling you to avoid twisted ankles and falls.

Your running shoe size often differs from your day shoe. If you find you get black or sore toenails after a run, it's a classic sign that your shoes don't fit properly. When you try shoes on, wear a pair of your usual cushioned, breathable running socks and make sure there's a thumb's width of space between your big toe and the end of the shoe when you're standing up. They should be neither too wide nor too narrow, and feel like an extension of your foot rather than a boat in which you slide around, or a vice in which your toes are squeezed like a row of tinned sardines.

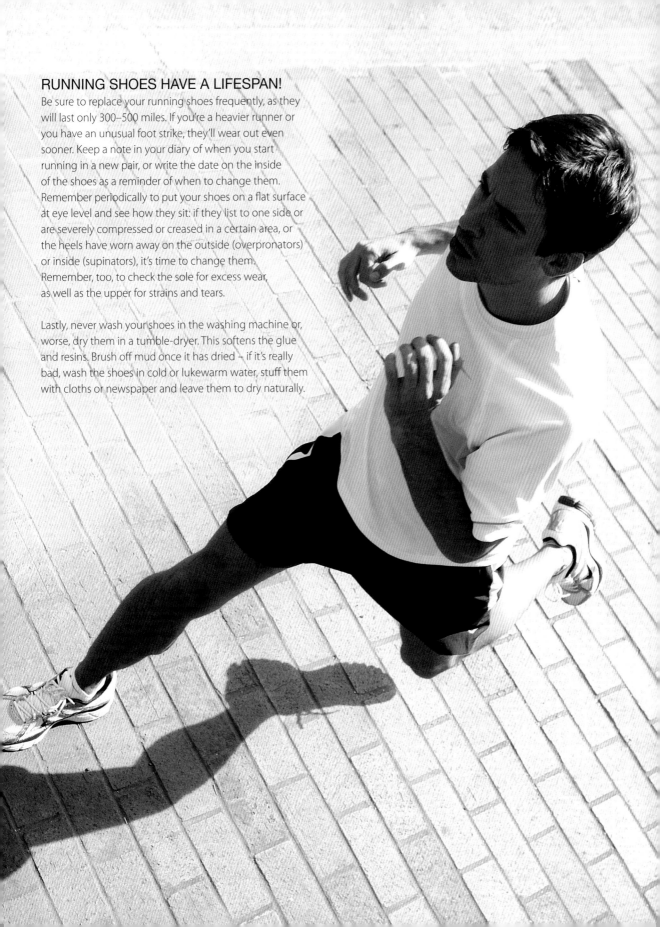

RUNNING SHOES HAVE A LIFESPAN!

Be sure to replace your running shoes frequently, as they
will last only 300–500 miles. If you're a heavier runner or
you have an unusual foot strike, they'll wear out even
sooner. Keep a note in your diary of when you start
running in a new pair, or write the date on the inside
of the shoes as a reminder of when to change them.
Remember periodically to put your shoes on a flat surface
at eye level and see how they sit: if they list to one side or
are severely compressed or creased in a certain area, or
the heels have worn away on the outside (overpronators)
or inside (supinators), it's time to change them.
Remember, too, to check the sole for excess wear,
as well as the upper for strains and tears.

Lastly, never wash your shoes in the washing machine or,
worse, dry them in a tumble-dryer. This softens the glue
and resins. Brush off mud once it has dried – if it's really
bad, wash the shoes in cold or lukewarm water, stuff them
with cloths or newspaper and leave them to dry naturally.

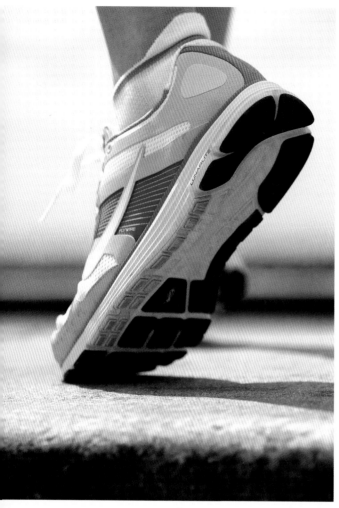

A running shoe basically consists of three sections: the outsole, the midsole and the upper. There are a few factors involved in the composition of the outsole that determine the traction of the shoe. These, in turn, determine whether it's for road-, trail-, or grass-running. Different compounds may be used that slightly alter the speed, force of impact and foot transition in order to get better performance on wet surfaces. A softer outsole, such as blown rubber, for example, will wear faster but give a bit more shock absorption and make for a slightly slower transition from landing to take-off.

The midsole is where the main characteristics of the shoe are located, and is where most of the shock absorption takes place. It's also where any anti-pronation or supination measures are found.

The upper is all about breathability, comfort and fit: the latest materials are used to ensure that the shoe is as light as possible and your foot is as well supported and cradled as it can be. A lot of research goes into the placing of the seams and the stitching so as to eliminate chafing. I remember the days when we were advised to wear in a new pair of shoes by walking around in them for a few days before running in them. That advice is now obsolete – you should be able to run in a good pair straight out of the box without any problems. Of course, it goes without saying that you always try out a new pair in training before you race in them, just in case.

anatomy of a running shoe

HEEL TAB
The part of the shoe that surrounds and protects the Achilles tendon, and helps lock the shoe around the heel.

EYELETS
The holes through which the laces are threaded. Extra top eyelets can improve the fit around the ankle.

MIDSOLE
Middle layer that provides cushioning between upper and outsole. Made from a shock-absorbing foam, it may include gel, air bags and other cushioning mechanisms.

TONGUE
Soft, padded, elongated flap that fits under the laces over the top of the foot to cushion it from pressure caused by the laces.

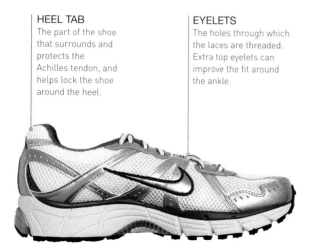

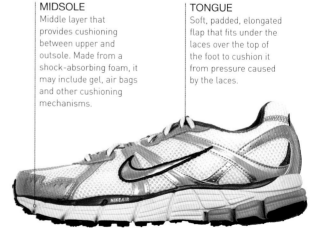

classic signs of foot discomfort

Pain across the top of the foot

Silly though it sounds, check that your laces aren't tied too tightly. You can also play around with the lacing pattern in the shoes to take the pressure off the top of your foot. If it remains a problem, look for a shoe with more padding in the tongue.

Tenderness in the arches or up your shins

This can be a sign that your arches are not getting enough support and that you are collapsing inwards as you run. Look for an anti-pronation shoe and consider adding some arch support in both your running and your walking shoes.

Chafing and soreness

Many companies manufacture shoes that cater for some of the more common problems. For example, the Nike women's Vomero has a softer, stretchy area in the upper beside the big toe that's designed to ease bunion symptoms. If you have any other problems, try a variety of different shoes to find the ones that feel the most comfortable. I'm not immune to these irritations: I have a small extra bone below the ankle bone on one foot that occasionally chafes and gives me discomfort if my shoes have a very rigid, high heel cup.

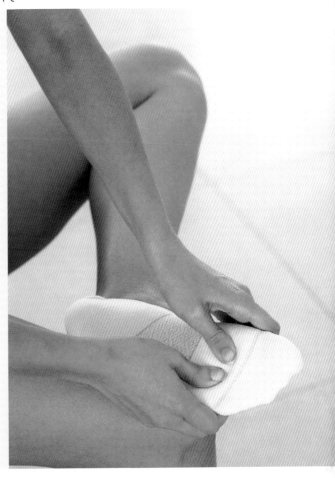

SOCKLINER
A removable insert that sits directly underneath the foot, designed to improve the shoe's fit.

UPPER
The part that encases the top of the foot. Made either from leather or synthetic material, it is breathable to allow heat to escape, keeping the foot cool.

FOOTBRIDGE
The firm material in the midsole that increases stability along the inner (arch) side of the shoe. Sometimes this is called the 'post'.

OUTSOLE
The durable under-surface of the shoe that provides traction on the ground. Reinforcing strips are overlaid at key stress points to help minimise impact.

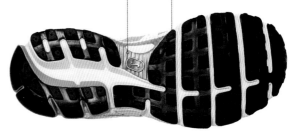

socks are important, too

When I consider all the carefully designed technical aspects of today's running-specific socks, I always think people are missing a trick when I see them being slung into shopping baskets as an afterthought.

After all, who would dream of running in a cotton T-shirt these days? The same advances in fabric technology that have so vastly improved our exercise clothing have also been applied to modern-day socks.

Apparel companies invest a lot of effort and research into socks that eliminate bulk and drag by studying the way the foot moves inside the shoe. Nike, for example, devotes enormous time and effort to observing runners on the track and on trails in order to pin down every last biomechanical factor that could possibly have a bearing on running comfort. Think of your sock as an important first layer of footwear that needs to work in harmony with your shoe, satisfying your individual requirements in cushioning, protection and support.

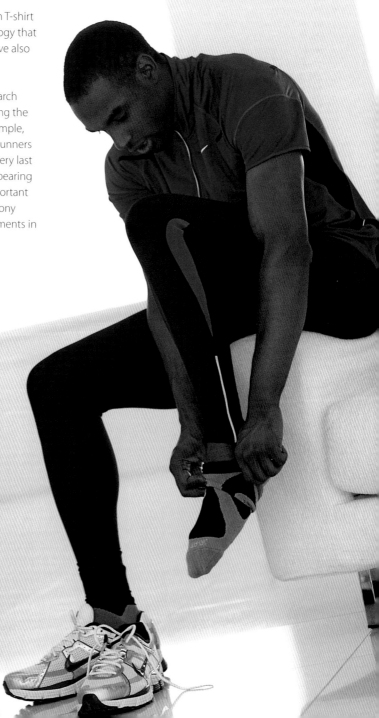

sock-buying considerations

Look out for special support features

- Pronators will find socks with areas designed to provide additional cushioning, as well as extra support in the arch and ankle area.
- Women may be more comfortable in socks designed specifically for them. Nike's research shows that women tend to blister in smaller areas – for example, a particular callus point on the inner edge of the ball of the foot. They also have greater flexibility in their toes, so a deeper toe box will accommodate this. A deeper heel will eliminate pull-down, especially with 'no show' socks.
- For runners who tend to roll over on their ankles, Nike's Structure sock gives increased arch and outer ankle ligament support.
- Double-layered socks have an added layer with extra anti-friction and anti-chafing properties, as well as giving additional cushioning around the ball of the foot.
- Compression socks are currently available in two versions:

Those that give extra support and warmth to the calf area, useful to runners prone to calf cramping and tightness in cold weather. They can also help speed recovery by assisting lymphatic drainage and blood flow from the lower limbs.

Medical-grade compression socks, such as the ones in which I like to race and do my long, hard training sessions. The theory is that by reducing muscle oscillation (vibration and impact forces through the calf muscle) you reduce capillary bleeding and micro-muscle fibre damage (the key causes of calf soreness), as well as muscle fatigue. I took part in research trials for these socks and can honestly say that I've never had sore calves after a marathon. Personally, I like to keep the socks on for a couple of hours afterwards to help with drainage and recovery.

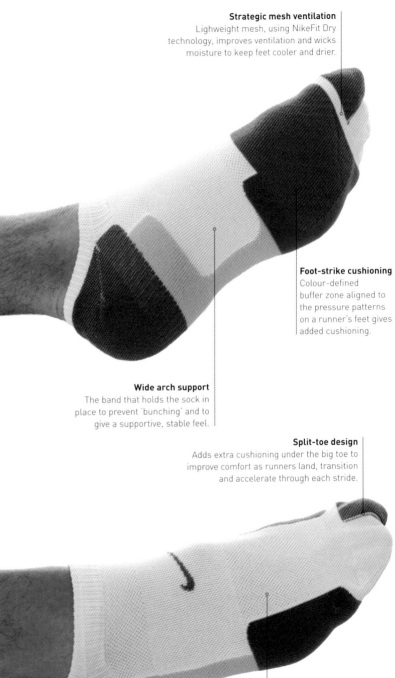

Strategic mesh ventilation
Lighweight mesh, using NikeFit Dry technology, improves ventilation and wicks moisture to keep feet cooler and drier.

Foot-strike cushioning
Colour-defined buffer zone aligned to the pressure patterns on a runner's feet gives added cushioning.

Wide arch support
The band that holds the sock in place to prevent 'bunching' and to give a supportive, stable feel.

Split-toe design
Adds extra cushioning under the big toe to improve comfort as runners land, transition and accelerate through each stride.

Anatomical left and right
Socks are designed specifically for the left and right foot to provide a natural fit.

Reinforced heel and toe
Ultra-durable construction in high-wear areas.

be aware of your posture

You may well say that I'm the last person to talk about posture, given my head-bobbing running style. Well, it's true that my head bobs, but it's as much a part of the way I run as Michael Johnson's upright, high-stepping sprint style when he was the world record-holder over 400m and 200m.

It hasn't held me back or given anyone cause for alarm in terms of potential damage. In fact, people recognise me, so I'm comfortable with it. If you cover my head and look at the rest of the way I run, my style is pretty economical, so my view is that the time and energy I'd need to spend trying to correct it just wouldn't be worth any gains.

However, there are a few postural skills that will make a real difference to your running efficiency:

Shoulders: Do you ever gradually become aware that your shoulders have crept up towards your ears? If you're like me, you do this subconsciously when you strain or get tired, which has the effect of tightening up everything else and costing you wasted energy. This slows you down. Try dropping your arms for a bit, or rolling your shoulders back a few times to get them down and more relaxed. Relaxed shoulders affect the way you hold your entire upper body all the way down to your hips, which, in turn, control the way you swing your arms. There is synergy between your shoulders and your lower body, which are connected through your abdomen and mid-section. For optimum performance, they need to work together, without tension. Besides, think of how much energy it takes to maintain tension in the body – what a waste this is when you need to be using every last drop to help you run.

Arm swing: When your shoulders are loose and low, your arms will hang naturally. Swing them at your sides from front to back, with more movement backwards than forwards; keep your fingers relaxed with a 90º angle at the

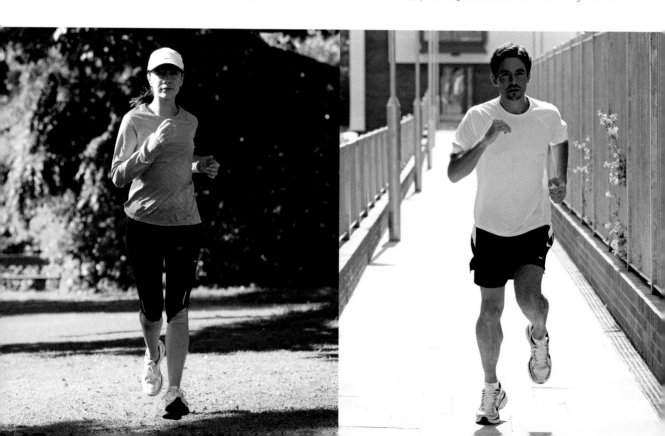

elbows. But try not to swing your arms across your body – this causes your torso to rotate from side to side around your spine, sapping your energy and slowing you down.

Upper body: The perfect running posture is leaning ever so slightly forwards from upright, with your spine straight and the angle between your straight back leg and bent lead leg approximately 80°–90°. By leaning forwards very slightly you maintain forward momentum as you run; this has the effect of giving you more energy and efficiency. Your eye line should be on the ground several metres in front of you, which is the natural angle of gaze. Obviously, you're not leaning so far forwards that you risk falling over. At the same time, never lean backwards as you run – this causes a braking action with each foot-strike, and as well as costing you time and energy, it imposes a lot of strain on your lower back, feet and ankles. Train yourself to maintain good spinal alignment. Treat yourself to a good osteopathic or chiropractic session every so often to help iron out the kinks.

Strike action: It's generally pretty difficult to change your strike action. The best thing is to make sure that your shoes and/or orthoses support your own individual strike action in the best way to optimise running efficiency. Generally, a midfoot or forefoot strike is a little more

efficient, especially at faster speeds. With both these styles of running, there's a shorter contact time with the ground and a faster, stronger toe-off. All the time that your foot is in contact with the ground, the energy of the foot strike is being absorbed into it, rather than being put back into your next stride.

Try to avoid over-striding, which puts excessive strain on your lower back and hamstrings. Your stride naturally lengthens when you run faster and shortens when you run uphill, but your cadence should generally remain much the same. A good way to measure your cadence is to count foot strikes per minute when you're running at a reasonable pace. Start with the first time the left foot strikes the ground and count every left strike for each minute. Repeat for the right foot. Left and right should be roughly the same. In very general terms, longer distance runners tend to have a higher cadence than shorter distance runners, making them more efficient as the distance goes on. Sprinters will have a higher knee lift and heel-to-bum movement than distance runners. My cadence is around 94. While it's a good idea to look at ways to slightly modify your stride action or make it a little more efficient, it's not an area that you should spend hours tearing your hair out over or over-analysing. If you feel relaxed when you run, then be happy with your style.

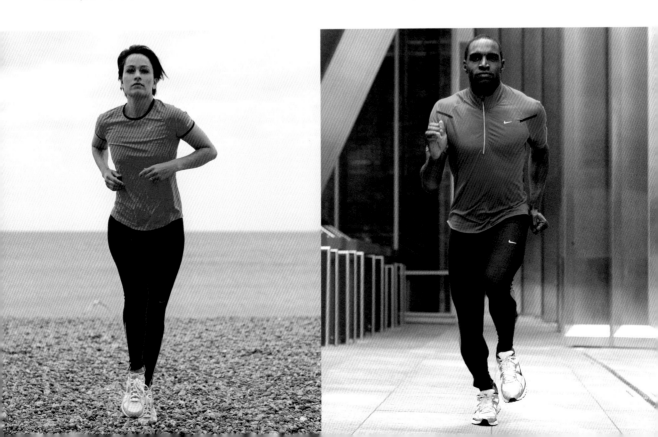

what to wear

There's a huge range of excellent-quality running apparel out there. You can take your chances wearing uncomfortable, stylish kit when you're out for a few hours on the town, but when you're running long distances you need optimal performance and support from your clothing.

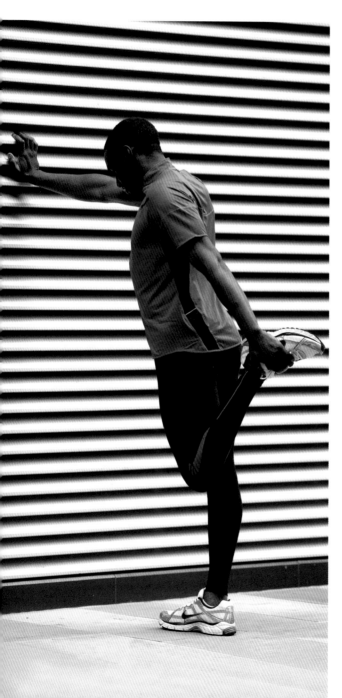

Luckily, sports companies devote a lot of time and effort to apparel design, so clothing can be stylish and feel great, as well as helping improve your performance and enjoyment. It all adds to the feel-good factor of running.

The key areas to look out for in all running clothing are:

Moisture management: The latest fabric technology is designed to wick moisture away from your body, ensuring you remain cool and dry in warm conditions and warm and dry in colder conditions. Unless you're still living in the dark ages, I doubt very much that you're running or exercising in cotton fabrics. But in case you still are, here's a fact to make you think again: cotton absorbs and then holds 8% of its weight in moisture; polyester (such as Dri-FIT) retains just 0.4% of its weight – besides, it's already far lighter to begin with. What's more, modern fabrics wash, dry and wear far more easily. When I'm travelling I can wash out Dri-FIT kit at night, shake it hard and hang it in the shower; by the morning it will be dry and look perfect.

Anti-chafing: Look out for streamlined garments that have as few seams as possible. Any excess bulk and areas of potential irritation need to be minimised to reduce the chances of chafing.

Optimal support and fit: Technical fabrics provide support where you need and want it without compromising on moisture management or feel. This is particularly important in chilly weather when you need extra warmth: high-tech fabrics can be layered without feeling bulky. The greatest research effort is carried out in women's apparel: a lot of testing and trialling goes into the production of the most effective sports bras and tops in order to ensure support for the wide variety of shapes and sizes. Nike recently conducted the widest study of the human body since World War II and then re-crafted its bodyfit criteria and sizing policy to more accurately reflect and accommodate our modern-day shapes.

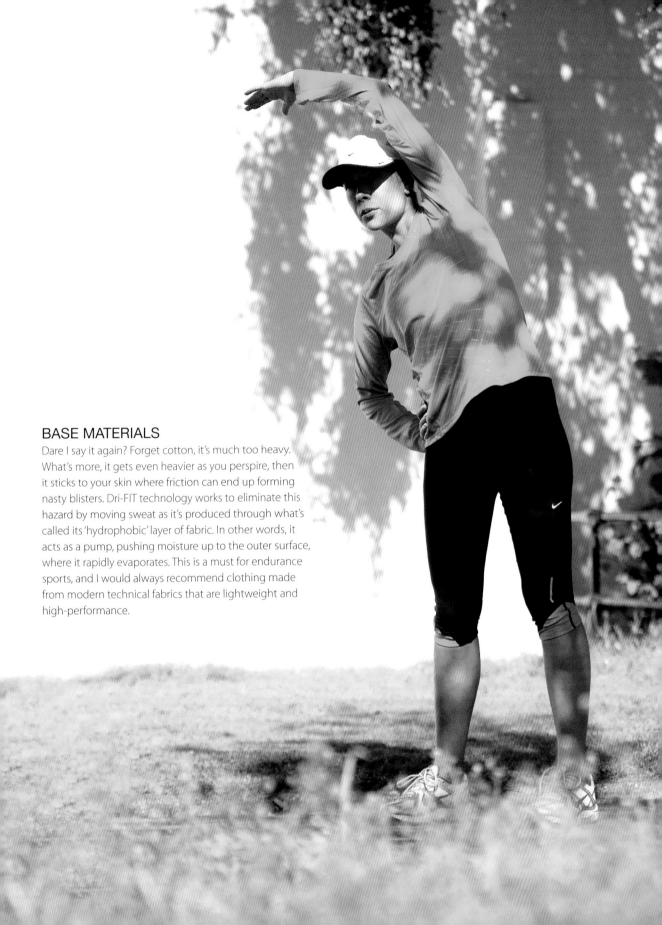

BASE MATERIALS

Dare I say it again? Forget cotton, it's much too heavy.
What's more, it gets even heavier as you perspire, then
it sticks to your skin where friction can end up forming
nasty blisters. Dri-FIT technology works to eliminate this
hazard by moving sweat as it's produced through what's
called its 'hydrophobic' layer of fabric. In other words, it
acts as a pump, pushing moisture up to the outer surface,
where it rapidly evaporates. This is a must for endurance
sports, and I would always recommend clothing made
from modern technical fabrics that are lightweight and
high-performance.

RUNNING IN WINTER

When the thermometer plummets, layer thinner fabrics that you can remove as you warm up, rather than wearing one single heavy layer. When you first step out through the door you should feel a little chilly, knowing that you'll be comfortable after a few minutes' running.

One thing that's important to bear in mind is that once you're exercising, your core will rarely be cold. The areas to think about are the extremities – your hands and ears/head. A great deal of research goes into producing gloves for different conditions: for sub-zero temperatures there's extra thickness, as well as special fabrics to protect areas that are more prone to wind chill and cold. I often race in lightweight gloves, because even when the rest of my body is warm, a slight chill can make my hands uncomfortable and divert my concentration. This can cause tension to travel up my arms into my body just when I want full control of my hands, especially in marathon races (no dropped drinks, thank you very much!).

Headwear is equally vital: your brain needs to be comfortable for you to perform optimally, so thermal hats and ear warmers can be a big help in the cold. I also love caps when I'm running in the rain: it keeps the water out of my eyes and off my head, making the going easier and giving a more pleasant experience.

Choose a jacket specifically designed for running: it needs to be water and wind resistant, lightweight, comfortable and to fit well enough that it never restricts movement, but also leaves no excess fabric flapping or rustling. Choose a top-quality, water-resistant yet breathable fabric such as Nike Storm-FIT. Clever use of air vents and openings in strategic places will allow it to breathe as you heat up. There's also a wide range of jacket/gilets with sleeves you can detach when you've warmed up, making buying and packing two separate jackets – one with sleeves and one without – unnecessary (one example is the Nike Shifter Jacket). A light-coloured, high-visibility fabric and/or reflective strips will allow motorists and cyclists to see you easily. It's a good idea to choose clothing with additional reflective features, as some of your runs are likely to be in the dark. An alternative is to wear reflective, fluorescent armbands – the latest have built-in flashing lights.

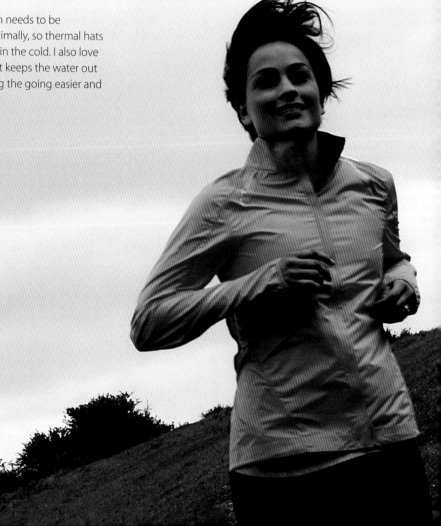

Think about what you like to take with you: mobile phone? Look for shorts or tights with a pocket. Keys and money? Look for a smaller key fob pocket to accommodate them snugly, cutting out annoying jangling as you run.

UNDERWEAR

What you wear underneath is just as crucial as what you wear on top. Men need to be concerned with chafing – the most commonly afflicted areas are the nipples and the groin.

Women have rather more to think about, given the more complicated nature of their anatomy. Chief among the necessary items is a well-fitting, high-impact sports bra, especially for larger breasted runners. This is vital for your back and upper body comfort, as the breast consists mainly of fatty tissue, mammary glands and muscle; the muscle, however, is too deep to be of much help. What little natural support there is comes from thin bands of connective tissue called Cooper's ligaments. So, to prevent drooping, always wear a proper sports bra. Most brands do a wide range, as well as cropped tops and vests with built-in support.

GARMENT CARE

There are certain recommended procedures that you need to follow in order to care for and maintain the performance of your garments.

Modern fabrics such as Dri-FIT and Storm-FIT should be washed with liquid detergents, but make sure you don't add fabric softener. Liquid detergents leave less residual dirt and oil on the fabrics during the wash cycle, especially with energy-saving water washes. Fabric softener should be avoided, as the silicone products coat the fabric fibres, destroying their moisture-management properties. However, you can tumble-dry these fabrics on a low heat setting, as this actually has the effect of lifting the fibres and restoring their properties. Indeed, if you find that your jacket is less water resistant than it used to be, put it through a water-only wash (no soap) and then tumble-dry to get the fluorocarbon chains functioning again – these give the jacket its water resistance properties. Don't over-dry the garment – it will just fill with static!

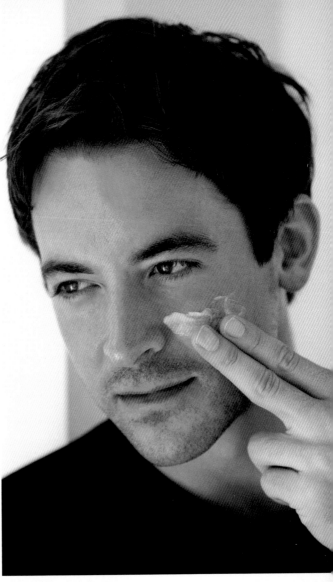

sun safety

Given the anti-ageing benefits of running, you don't want to negate them by failing to protect your skin. We tend to remember to slap on sun cream in summer, but forget it when we're at higher altitudes where the air feels cooler on the skin. Yet ultraviolet rays are more intense and more damaging up there, even when it's cloudy. Choose a lotion or sports spray and use them all year round. Take note of the SPF, and make sure they're water and sweat resistant, but still allow your skin to breathe. Don't skimp on the key areas for runners: shoulders, back of the calves, tops of the ears and bridge of the nose, as well as the crown of the head (especially if you're thin on top). It needs to be easy to apply so that you'll use it regularly, and it should smell agreeable, as the aroma will become stronger as you sweat.

gadgets and gizmos

These may be considered as non-essential by some – indeed, you don't need them in order to run – but I've found that they can enhance my running experience enormously.

Running sunglasses: These aren't just a fashion statement (although it is important that you like the look and feel good wearing them), they serve a functional purpose by allowing your face to relax as you run. Once you allow the tension in by squinting, you cost yourself energy and risk headaches and a stiff, sore neck and shoulders. Moreover, they protect your eyes from grit and debris and are a real help during allergy season. A good pair of running sunglasses will be lightweight and won't bounce, pinch the bridge of your nose, or press down hard on the tops of your ears. Moreover, they come with different styles of lenses to suit the conditions in which you most frequently run. For example, you can get lenses that cut out reflective brightness from road surfaces, reduce exceptional glare, or adapt quickly to changing light conditions when you run through trees. They also cope well with heat build-up and have special anti-fogging features. Ask the sales person for an explanation of the key functions and try out several pairs to be sure that they feel comfortable before you buy.

Heart rate monitor: This very useful device measures how fast your heart is beating and, using this information, feeds back the level of intensity you're putting/not putting into your run. You strap it around your chest, put a drop of moisture on the monitoring device and position it just over your heart, where it 'listens' to your heartbeat. The monitor comes with a watch to which it transmits the information gathered as you run: number of heartbeats per minute, how far you have run, how long you have been running and, of course, the time – all easily viewable on your wrist. Wearing a heart monitor allows you to check your progress while you're running. Data of this quality enables you to be specific in your training and make sure that your runs and other exercise sessions are achieving what you set out to do. (See Chapter 5: Raising your game, for more detailed information.) The top-end monitors are also available with an interface that allows you to download your data on to your computer, and then review how it went.

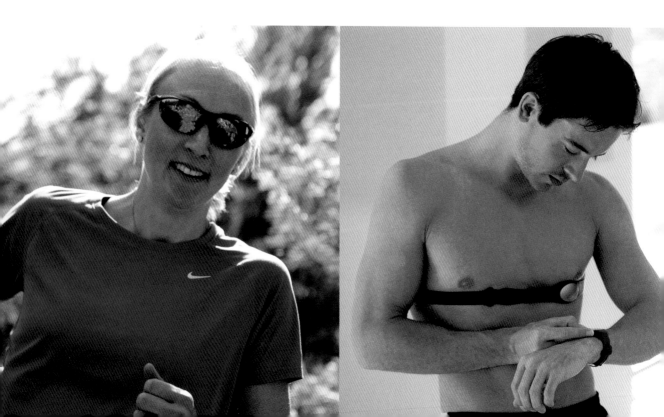

MP3 player or iPod: Many people prefer to run to music. Indeed, it has actually been proved that an upbeat tempo can improve performance. For my marathon preparation, I put together a playlist that I listen to before the race to remind myself how the training has gone. During some marathons I've actually occasionally heard songs from my playlist from pubs and bands along the route – this has helped produce my fastest mile splits for the same perceived effort. I tend to enjoy music when I'm running on the treadmill or cross-training in the gym, and on tired days I do find that it helps to tune into inspirational beats. But as a rule, I prefer to run outdoors without it, in tune with my surroundings and feelings. There are those who are surgically attached to their iPods and there are purists who see music only as a distraction; in between, most people mix it up as they please. Obviously, don't let music drown out what's going on around you, blunting your awareness and reactivity. Switch off in noisy traffic and when you're running alone in quiet areas.

If you're among those who enjoy running with music, the Nike+ system is a really good idea. It consists of an iPod Nano and a sensor that you put into a built-in pocket under the insole of Nike running shoes. Calibrate it initially by running a measured distance in the shoes; after this it's incredibly accurate and will give you your pace, the distance you've covered and your average speed – all while continuing to play your favourite music! And I love this bit: you can programme it to play a 'power song' at the touch of a button if you're going through a tough patch and need an additional boost. There's also a range of clothing made by Nike into which you can slot your iPod. This enables you to run without the hassle of wires flapping around you, or worrying about it unclipping from your waistband.

power songs

how to choose them

Music is a useful way to help you run at a consistent pace and give you a lift. However, it takes time to compile a playlist: each track has to have just the right beat to match your desired speed or to help you increase your pace. Too much James Blunt and you'll still be running when the others are already showered and heading for breakfast. But if you play unrelentingly fast tracks too early on, you'll end up running out of steam and/or sustaining an injury.

The easier option is to check out the playlists on www.nikeplus. com, which are designed to help you pace yourself over your chosen distance.

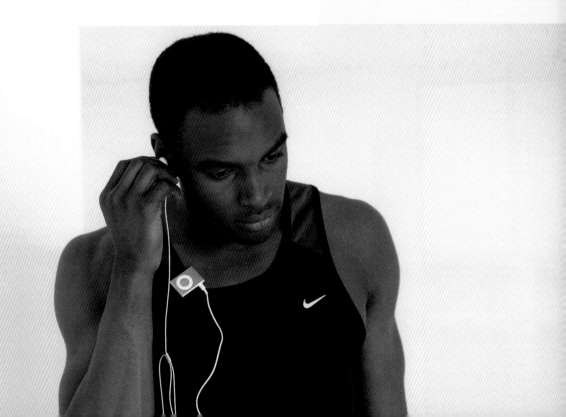

3 taking care of your body

Once you know how to keep your muscles, joints and ligaments well tuned, your body will live up to even the most exacting expectations.

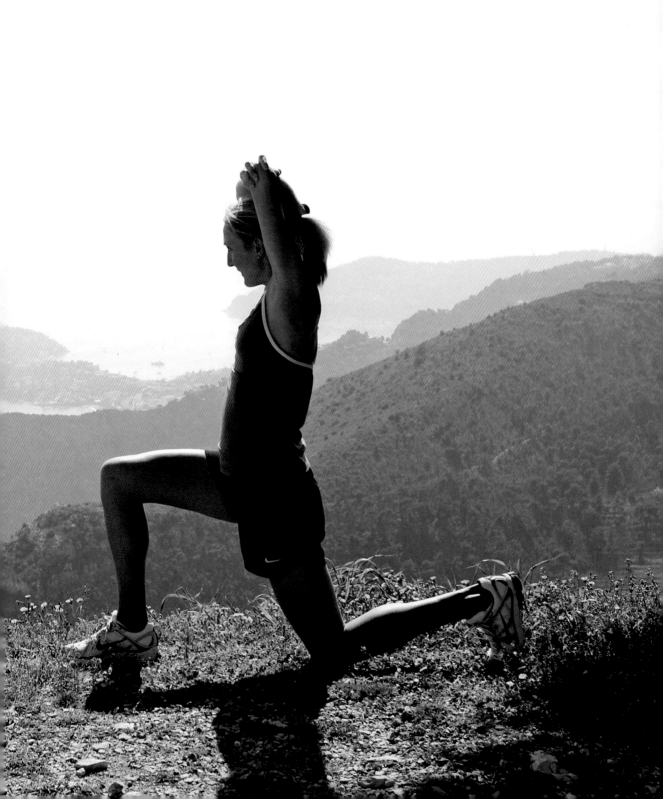

getting results from your efforts

Your body is your best friend and No.1 tool. Listen to it and treat it with respect and care, and it will serve you well.

You can only expect your body to perform if you maintain it. Abuse it by not fuelling it, not doing preventative work or not heeding the first signs of trouble, and you will struggle. At worst, it will break down completely. This chapter deals with how to prepare and care for your body mechanically.

WARMING UP

For runners of all levels and distances, warming up the joints and muscles is essential to preventing injury. It prepares the body for the demands of the training session or race and enables you to work at optimum efficiency. Joints contain synovial fluid – a bit like lubricating oil for loosening stubborn locks or creaky hinges. Our joints are similar: when they are cold, the synovial fluid is thick and sticky and the joints sluggish. Once warm, it's loose and less viscous, allowing the joints to glide smoothly. Generally, the shorter the distance, the longer the warm-up. Sprinters have to unleash explosive power the instant they propel themselves out of the blocks, so they spend at least an hour warming up. But distance runners' muscles also need to be warm and pliable, the body lightly sweating but not fatigued, and the heart rate slightly raised before they set off.

In hot weather, 5–7 minutes of jogging followed by some good stretching and a few strides should be enough. In normal conditions, I like to warm up by slowly jogging for 12–15 minutes and then stretching thoroughly with dynamic and resisted stretches. I finish off with controlled strides. Warm muscles stretch better, and an initial easy jog gives me a good indication of which areas I need to concentrate on when I'm stretching.

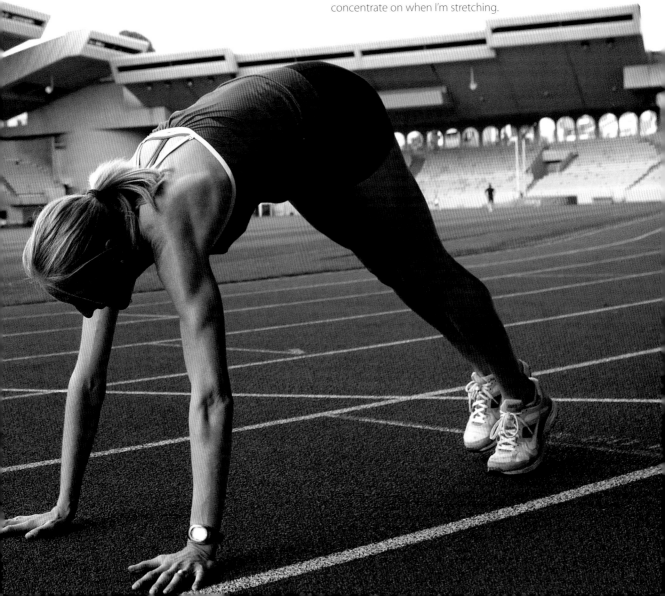

pre-run static stretching

Spend 10–15 seconds on each stretch. Approach them gently, as your muscles haven't yet warmed up.

1 open the chest
Extend your arms wide to the side at shoulder height until your shoulder blades squeeze together behind you.

2 loosen the hips
Rotate the pelvis – imagine you're trying to keep a hula-hoop circling your waist. Push your bum out backwards and your pelvis forwards as you rotate, so that your hips perform as big a circle as possible.

3 loosen your shoulders
Windmill your arms slowly from back to front and then front to back. Progress by moving them in alternate directions.

4 loosen the spine
Hands on hips, rotate the torso to one side, then the other.

5 stretch your calves
To stretch the bulging section of the calf (gastrocnemius), place your palms flat against a wall just below shoulder height and position the leg you want to stretch about 4ft back from the wall. The heel is flat on the ground and the leg straight. Your front leg is halfway between your back leg and the wall, knee bent. With back straight, lean forward until you feel the calf stretch. To stretch the lower calf (soleus) where the leg joins the ankle, maintain this posture and bend your back leg until you feel the stretch.

6 loosen your side muscles
Stand with your legs slightly wider than hip-width apart. With palms facing inwards, bend slowly to the left, running your hand down the leg towards your knee. Now bend to the right. Keep your spine straight – don't allow yourself to bend forward.

7 quad stretch
To stretch the front of the thigh, stand with knees together, grasp a foot with the same-side hand and, keeping your hips forward, gently pull it into the bum. If you don't feel anything, push your hips forward a bit more.

8 loosen your knees
Squat, keeping your back flat and straight and your thighs as close to parallel to the ground as you can while still maintaining good form.

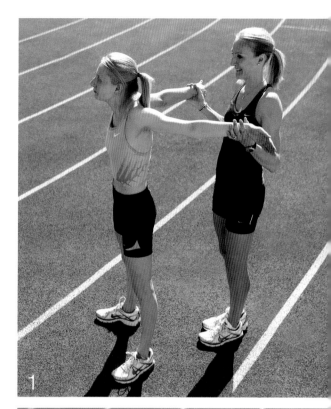

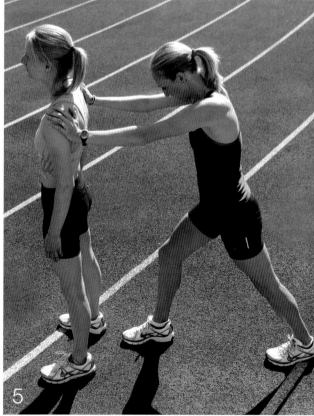

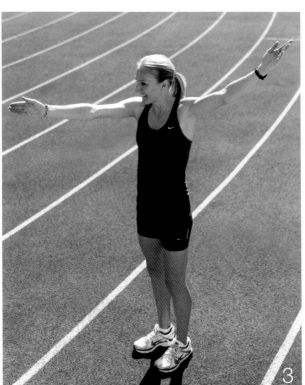

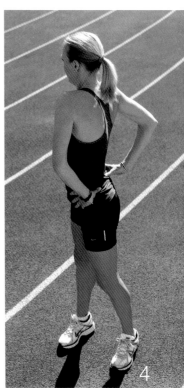

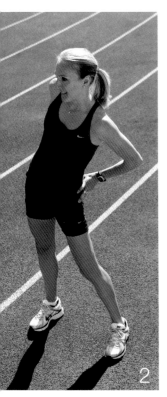

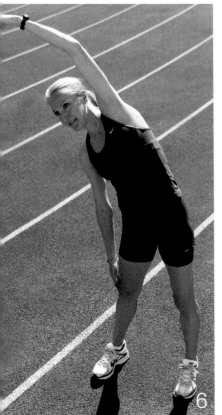

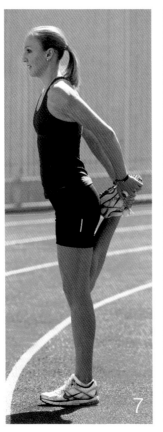

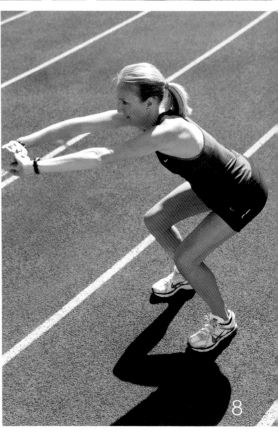

pre-run dynamic stretching

After your warm-up jog, when your joints are lubricated and your muscles ready, spend 30–60 secs on each of these.

1 crossovers
Take small sideways steps to the left by placing one foot behind the other, then switch legs and reverse the pattern coming back. Your hips will swivel slightly.

2 side-walking lunges
Take three hops to the right and, with legs wide apart, lunge to the right – your right leg will be bent to about 90°, and your left leg will be straight out to the side. Now take three hops to the left and do likewise. This stretches the adductor muscles of the groin and inside thigh.

3 walking straight-leg kicks
Walk forwards, kicking alternate legs straight up in front of you to waist height to touch the opposite hand.

4 walking knee raises
Raise each knee alternately and hug it as close to your chest as possible, then step forward and repeat with the other leg. Concentrate on maintaining good balance and keeping your hips high and forward.

5 walking lunges
Step forward with alternating legs, each time dropping your back knee to just above the ground, creating a 90° angle at the front knee. Keep your torso upright (don't lean forwards) and make sure the knee of your lead foot doesn't travel in front of your toes – this imposes too much strain on the knee.

6 bum kicks
Walking backwards, at each step bend the knee and alternately raise each foot behind you until it touches the bum, activating the hamstrings and glutes.

7 side-to-side hip swings
Holding on to a post, swing each leg 10 times in turn from the hip out to each side, back and forth, side to side.

8 forward-back hip swings
Repeat the hip swing as above, this time swinging your leg up forwards to stretch the hamstring and then back, fully, to activate the glutes. Concentrate on keeping your hips stable.

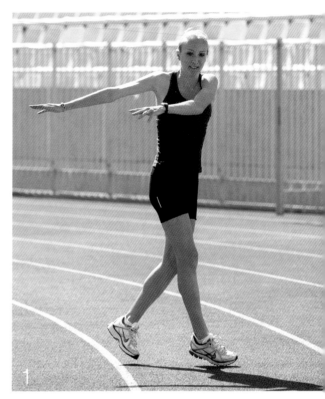

1

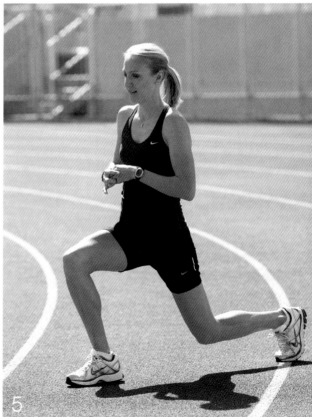

5

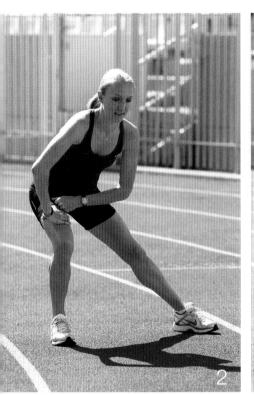

2

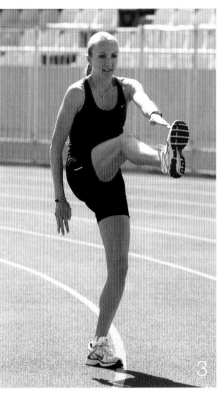

3

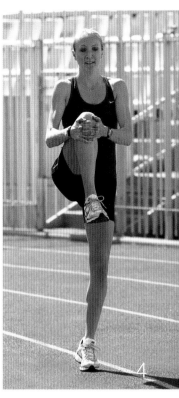

4

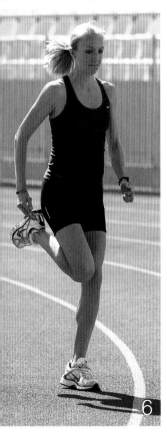

6

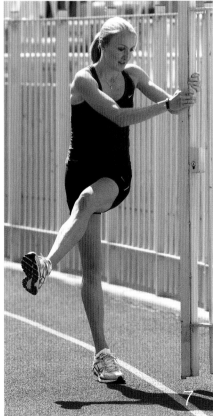

7

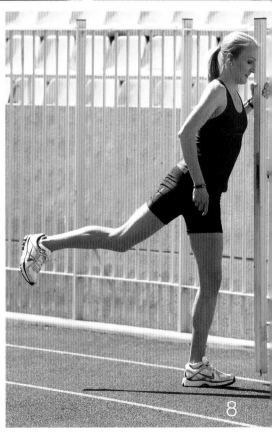

8

POST-RUN STRETCHES

Think of the stretching you do after you've finished your run as an integral part of it: if you leave it out, your training session is, quite simply, incomplete. There's good, solid common sense behind this assertion and you can pay a high price for ignoring it.

We stretch to increase our flexibility – i.e. to increase the distance our muscles allow our limbs to move before the muscles start straining – and also to aid recovery. By working at lengthening the muscles after exercise, we achieve three vital results: we improve their range of movement and increase their dynamic power while they are still warm; we reduce muscle fatigue and assist the process of repair; and we help prevent injury and alleviate muscle soreness.

High-intensity exercise, or taking up exercise again after a lay-off, brings with it an all-too-familiar feeling a day or two later. How often have you tried to leap out of bed with your customary *joie de vivre* only to collapse, groaning, back into it? Thank you, DOMS (Delayed Onset of Muscle Soreness) – the tiny tears in the muscle fibres, together with the accumulated waste products that have built up in your muscles during exercise.

Areas of particular importance to runners are the Achilles tendons, calves, hamstrings and iliotibial bands (see 'Symptoms to look out for' on page 62). Tightness in these areas is an occupational hazard, but allowing them to get even tighter can lead to tears, or knee and hip problems. This can only be prevented or alleviated by stretching.

8 points to remember about stretching

1   Stretching is a highly individual experience: no two runners will be able to stretch to the same extent, since one person's flexibility will always be greater or less than the next. Distance runners are famously among the least flexible of all, which is why we, especially, need to work on it every day.

2   Only stretch when your muscles are warm, i.e. stretch immediately after running. Once they have started to cool down, you'll be stretching resistant muscles, which could tear. Never force a stretch.

3   It takes six seconds for the stretch reflex to kick in, so holding a stretch for anything less than 20 seconds isn't worth doing. Hold for as long as a minute when your muscles are very tight.

4   Never bounce up and down during a static (stationary) stretch: get into the stretch position and hold it for 20–30 seconds.

5   Stretch only to the point where you can feel tension in the muscle. Muscles are designed to stretch no more than 1.6 times their length at the most – indeed, asking even this much flexibility will make a muscle recoil to prevent it tearing, potentially incurring pulls and strains.

6   Remember to breathe while you're holding a stretch! Not as daft as it sounds – runners sometimes do unconsciously hold their breath.

7   It's worth having a rope with you – I carry mine everywhere, because I need it to properly stretch my hamstrings, glutes and quads on my own.

8   For really tight – even painfully tight – muscles, self-massage with a foam roller (a massage ball or tennis ball works well too) is very worthwhile. The technical name for this is 'myofascial release', and it's worth asking someone with experience of applying it how to do this properly. The basic method involves locating the area of tightness, a.k.a. the 'trigger point', and placing the foam roller/ball directly underneath it so that the weight of the limb bears down on it. Roll the limb over it, stopping at particularly tight areas; roll up and down 10–15 times, gradually working into and releasing the tightness.

So, with these words of wisdom ringing in your ears, what are the best post-run stretches we can do to help guard against misfortune?

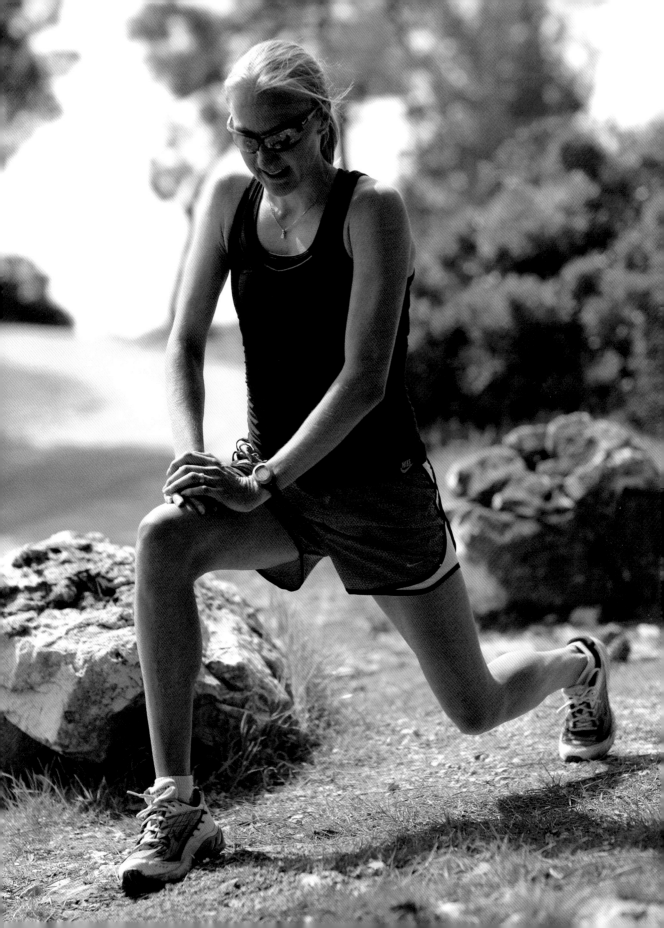

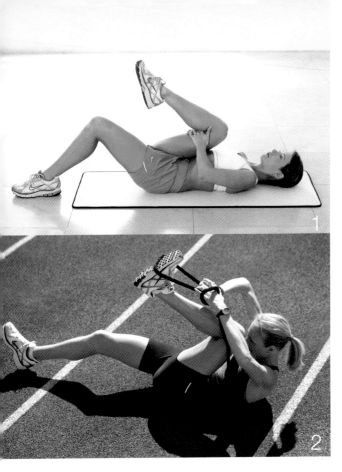

hamstring stretch

The hamstrings are three muscles at the back of each thigh, notoriously inflexible in distance runners. The convenient way to do this is by putting a foot on a park bench or low wall and leaning forward from the hips, with your back flat, until you feel the stretch in the back of the thigh. Make sure your hips are level and facing forwards.

Alternative 1: If it's not cold and wet outdoors, lie on your back with your knees bent to 90°, feet on the ground. Raise one leg and, keeping the knee slightly bent, grasp it with both hands just below the knee and gently pull it towards your chest. Carefully straighten the knee a little to deepen the stretch. Repeat for the other leg.

Alternative 2: Using a rope, sit on the floor and loop it around the toes of the leg you're stretching. Lie back and, with a slight bend at the knee, pull the rope towards you, stretching the attachment to the bum. Then straighten the leg and pull the rope towards you to stretch the hamstrings. Finally, pull the rope out to the side and back towards you, stretching the adductors (groin muscles) and hamstrings; then back across your body and upwards to stretch the iliotibial band and abductors.

hip (piriformis) stretch

The piriformis muscle controls the outwards rotation of the hip. Keeping it in good order is particularly important for sports such as tennis and football, which require players to be able to change direction quickly. But even for runners consistently moving in a forward direction, a flexible piriformis muscle is important for a smooth running action and a stable pelvis.

Lie on your back and lift your knees to 90°, then cross your legs so that one ankle sits on the other knee. Grasp the leg that's hooked underneath and pull the knee towards your chest until you feel the stretch in your buttocks and hips. Now pull it out to the left and then to the right. Repeat for the other side.

Alternative: I often vary this by using the rope (see left): lie back and hook it around your foot, bend your knee back to your chest, straighten it and pull it across your body, feeling the stretch in the glutes and piriformis.

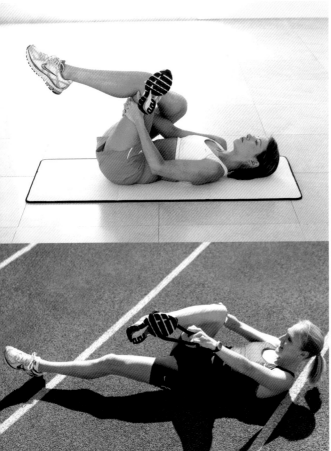

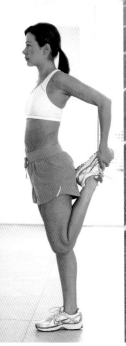

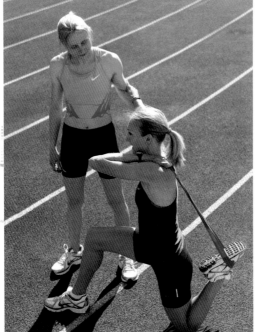

quadriceps stretch

The quads run down the front of the thigh and connect to the knee. The largest is the rectus femoris – it enables you to lift your knee and, because it connects to the pelvis, flex your hip. To keep it in good order, stand up straight, grasp one foot behind you and ease it towards your bum. Keep the knees together, pelvis level and hips forward. If you can't feel the stretch, push your hips further forward still.

Alternative: Kneel with one knee on a pad and the other foot in front. With pelvis level and glutes tightly squeezed, loop the rope around your toes, bring it over your shoulder and pull your foot towards your bum.

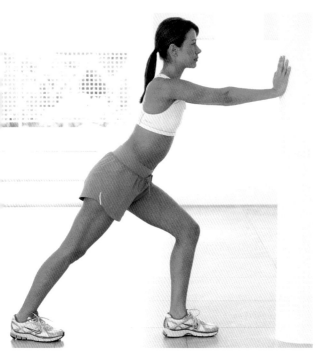

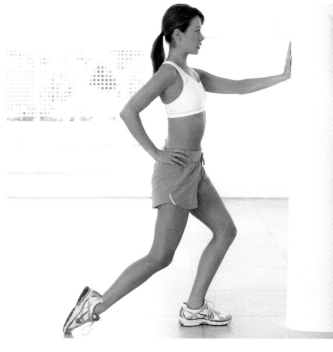

calf stretch

The calf muscle consists of the bulging gastrocnemius and the narrow soleus where the leg joins the ankle. They propel you as you run, and ache if you don't stretch. With palms on the wall just below shoulder height, place the leg to be stretched about 4ft from the wall, heel down and leg straight. The front leg is bent, halfway between your back leg and the wall. With back straight, lean forward until you feel the stretch in your calf. Now bring your back leg a bit closer to the wall, bend it and feel the stretch in your lower calf muscle.

shin stretch

This is a useful way of helping to keep the dreaded shin splints at bay (for more information on shin splints, see page 63). Stand up straight and extend one foot behind you so that the tops of your toes are facing downwards on the ground. Push the ankle towards the ground.

Alternative: Place your foot behind you on a bench or low wall and push down, as before. Massaging with a stick roller will also help to loosen the muscles.

strength training

Strength complements speed. You need it towards the end of a long run when you feel as though you're running on empty and need to maintain good form. And yet I talk to many fellow runners who worry that lifting weights will cause them to bulk up and hinder their running action.

They believe that in order to run further faster, they need to do yet more running to improve their performance. But imagine how they'd feel if they could increase their power and efficiency to enable them to burn off the guys on their shoulder in a sprint finish or even just lessen the effects of fatigue in a particularly gruelling race. You use your entire body to get you through a run, not just your legs, so don't neglect the rest of you.

A properly targeted weights programme will help make your muscles stronger and more resilient, but won't make you heavy or bulky. To some extent, this depends on your natural body type: an ectomorph (i.e. slightly built and light-boned) could lift quite heavy weights every day and never develop massive muscle bulk. However, this doesn't mean that if you have a heavier frame you shouldn't train with weights at all – your training should be appropriate to your build, which means using lighter weights and performing more repetitions per set.

It's not necessary to be a gym member to follow an effective strength training regime. You can strengthen your muscles using your own body weight; you can also use portable equipment at home such as a mat, rubber tube, Swiss ball, a range of dumbbells and a couple of different weights of medicine balls.

Of course, the wider range of facilities you'll usually find in a gym can be helpful. These may variously include swimming pools, bikes and cross-trainers, as well as barbells and kettle bells, fixed-weight machines and cables. In the end, where and how you choose to do your strength and conditioning work is a matter of choice.

The answer to strength training for runners doesn't lie in bench-pressing the equivalent of your own body weight. On the contrary, it needs to be functional and sport-specific. For distance runners, this means endurance-oriented and focused on movements that mimic those required by the sport. These will strengthen the muscles that power the actions demanded of you when you're running.

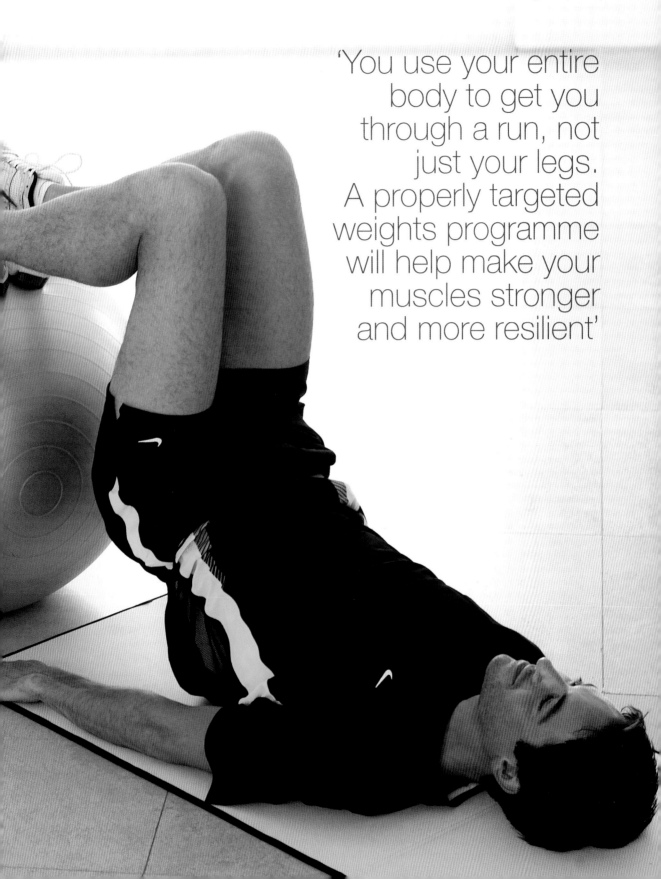

'You use your entire body to get you through a run, not just your legs. A properly targeted weights programme will help make your muscles stronger and more resilient'

4 IMPORTANT POINTS TO REMEMBER

In my experience, there are four points worth flagging up:

1 You may well believe that your legs are getting quite enough exercise already, given the mileage they're doing. Not true. In addition to training your upper body, you still need to work your lower body muscles. Making the muscles stronger helps them stay efficient for longer and speeds recovery, while reducing injury risk. Think about it: stronger, well-trained muscles are far more likely to be able to maintain good form and correct position as you tire. This means you'll be able to continue running strongly and efficiently for longer.

The other compelling reason for adopting a weight training routine is that glycogen (the fuel you need for energy when running) is stored in the muscles. It stands to reason, then, that the larger the percentage of muscle in relation to your total body mass, the bigger your fuel store and the better equipped you are for a long run or race.

2 Do your strength training programme two to three times a week, making sure to leave at least one full day between sessions to allow enough time to repair and develop the muscles that have been worked. Be warned: if you try to train with weights every day, you'll exhaust your muscles and weaken them rather than strengthen them. Once they have been stressed hard, your muscles need at least 48 hours in order to respond, recover and get stronger. The only major muscles in your body that you can safely work hard daily are your abdominals.

3 Make sure you perform each exercise through the full range of movement: this allows the muscle to strengthen all the way along the maximum range of expansion and contraction. It's a waste of time spending ages doing exercises if you're not working your muscles correctly.

4 Good technique (or 'form') is crucial. If you're a member of a gym, ask an instructor to demonstrate how the strength training exercises in this chapter should be performed so that you get it right from the word go. If you're not a gym member, ask someone with experience to show you. Besides the fact that sloppy technique reduces effectiveness, it can also be dangerous. Pay attention to the following recommendations and you'll be a textbook example of good weight-lifting technique:

- Keep your abdominal muscles braced at all times: pull your navel in towards your spine to support your back.
- Find your 'neutral spine' position by tilting your pelvis under and tucking in your tailbone, bringing your spine into alignment. This prevents the lower back from sagging, creating a point of weakness. When you check your posture sideways in a mirror, you should be straight from neck to hip, each vertebra stacked one above the other, the spine neither caving inwards nor bulging outwards.
- Keep your shoulders down: head off the creep towards your ears before it happens. Tension starts in the shoulders, but spreads like wildfire through the body.
- Breathe correctly: exhale during the most strenuous part of the movement (the drive phase); inhale during the easiest part (the release phase, when you're returning the weights to the starting position).
- Don't rush the movement: the more you slow it down, the greater the challenge. Fight the urge to release the weights quickly as soon as you've reached the most strenuous point in the movement – releasing slowly keeps the muscles loaded with tension for longer, giving the exercise greater intensity and enabling you to get the most out of it.

Your programme should be 'progressive' and 'periodised'. This is just shorthand for 'build up your strength and fitness over a specified period of time in order to achieve your goals by a given deadline'. For instance, if you wanted to get in shape in time for an August island-hopping trip in the Caribbean, you'd start working on yourself in early April to look buff in four months' time. Runners training for a specific event do likewise in order to arrive at race day in peak condition. (See 'Raising your game' on page 80 and 'Getting serious' on page 100.) Generally, we start with a broad and varied base programme, progressing to a more focused, harder and heavier lifting phase, finishing with a lighter, more explosive tapering phase timed to be ready just before an upcoming competition.

Consider having a strength assessment by a professional. For example, the muscles around my scapulae can be weak, causing my shoulders to hike up as I tire, so I make sure I strengthen them. Similarly, my hamstrings are weaker in comparison to my quads, so I work these slightly more. Also, a strong core and strong feet are hugely important for all runners, so these need to be worked on regularly.

core strength training programme

You can do this core programme two to three times a week at home with a Swiss ball, a dumbbell or medicine ball, a rope and an exercise band. I like to do it after an easy run when my muscles are warm but I'm not too tired.

If you're occasionally short of time, you don't need to do each one of these exercises at every single session, but make sure you do at least four of the abdominal (abs) ones, as well as the mini glutes circuit on page 53.

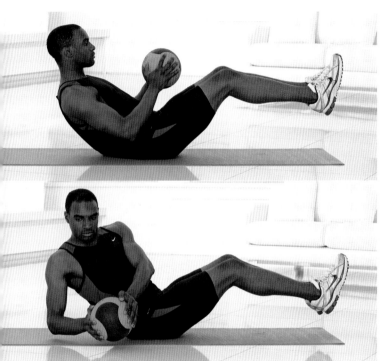

1 medicine ball twists
(10 reps each side)
Seated on a mat with your knees slightly bent, feet off the ground and lower legs parallel to the floor. Twist your torso to the right and touch the medicine ball to the floor beside you; then twist to the left and repeat. Make sure your arms aren't doing all the work – they are only following your torso as it twists from side to side.

Alternative: Sitting a little more upright, with knees slightly bent and feet off the ground, twist to the right to place the medicine ball directly behind your back; then twist to the left and pick it up, taking it across your front to the right to place it behind you again.

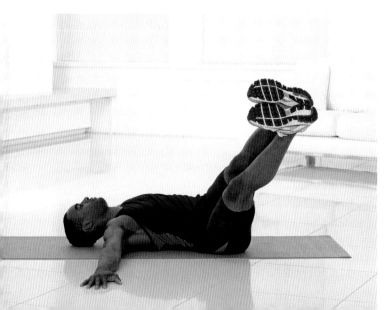

2 windscreen wipers
(8 to each side x 1–2 sets)
Lift both legs as close to 90° as you can manage. Keeping your feet together and legs straight, slowly lower them to the left and then the right (like windscreen wipers) as far as you can go while still keeping your hips on the floor. Extend your arms out to the sides for balance, if necessary.

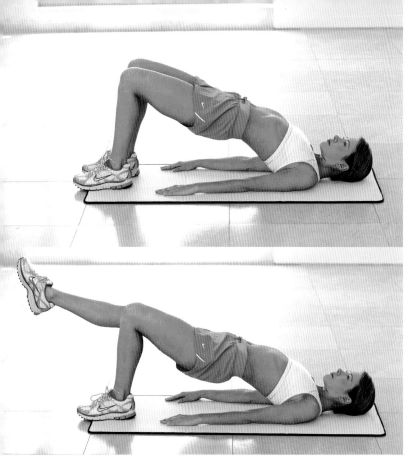

3 hip bridge
(6–10 reps each side x 2–3 sets)

With shoulders and feet on the floor and glutes squeezed, lift the hips up into a bridge. Hold your body in a straight line from shoulders to knees. Alternately raise and fully extend each leg, keeping them level with the body, then lower again, all the while maintaining a high, strong bridge.

Progression: Alternating legs, lower your pelvis to the floor and lift it up again between each rep, keeping the leg fully extended throughout. Make sure you use only the hips to lift and lower – your leg follows the hips, otherwise it's motionless. (Try to keep the toes of the raised foot pulled back towards your knee.)

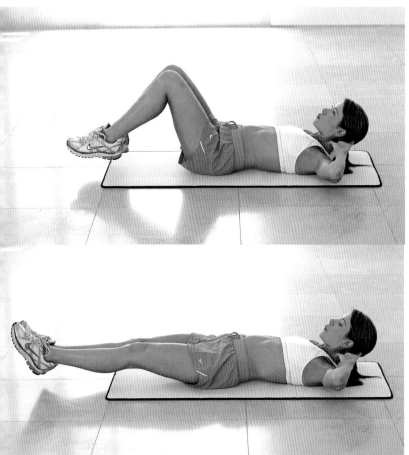

4 lying double foot slide
(10–15 reps x 1–2 sets)

Lying on your back with your knees at 90° and your feet an inch off the floor, slowly slide your feet away from you until your legs are fully extended. Lace your fingers behind your head and lift your shoulders slightly so that your back remains flat to the floor throughout. If you can't extend your legs fully while keeping your back flat on the floor, go only as far as you can for now; you'll be able to extend them further as you get stronger. Bring them slowly back in again and repeat.

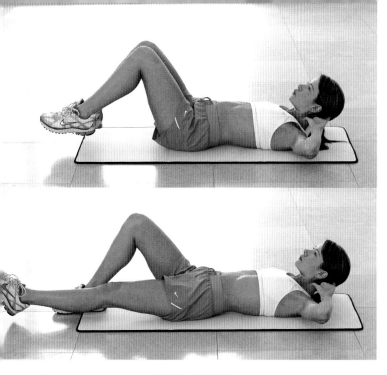

5 lying single-leg alternate slide
(10-15 each side x 1-2 sets)
Perform this exactly as in Exercise 4, but
this time doing it with just one leg at a
time. Again, go only as far as you can while
keeping your back flat on the floor.

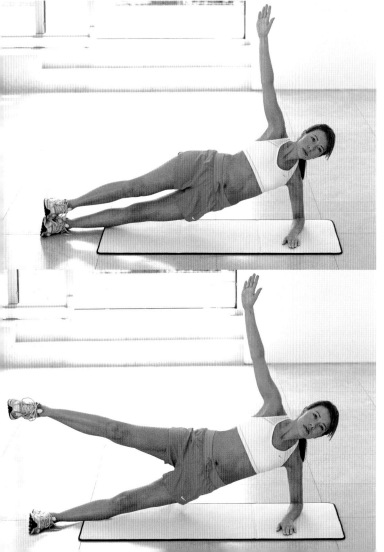

6 side plank
(hold for 30–60 secs)
Turn on to your side, so that your body is at
90° to the floor from head to toe, one foot
stacked on top of the other. Make sure that
your head is aligned with your spine – don't
allow it to hang forward. Hold, not allowing
your hip to dip towards the floor, then
repeat on the other side. Build up to the
point where you can do this side plank plus
the full plank on page 53 without coming
down in between.

Progression: Try lifting the top leg. Start
by just lifting it for 3–5 seconds at a time,
coming down in between. Gradually extend
the number of seconds until you can keep it
aloft for the duration of the exercise without
your hip sagging towards the floor.

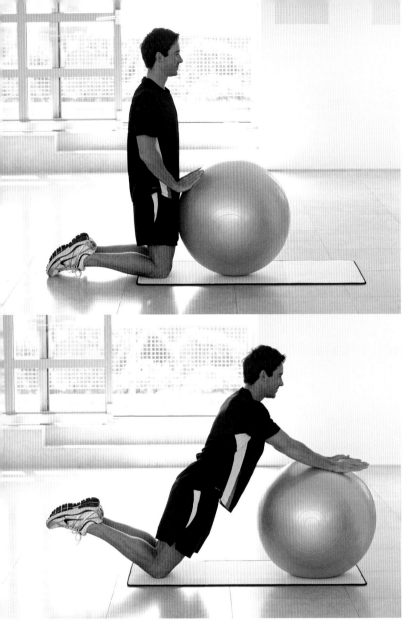

7 swiss ball roll-outs
(10 reps x 1 set)

Kneeling on the ground, with palms on the ball on the side nearest your body, squeeze your glutes hard and draw in your abs so that your body is straight and taut like a plank of wood. Pivoting on your knees, roll the ball forwards as far as possible until your arms are fully extended, using your strong and stable abs to prevent your lower back from sagging. Roll the ball back towards you using your triceps (the muscles at the back of your upper arms) keeping the bum tucked in and not allowing it to stick out.

Progression: Try doing the roll-out with one arm only. Use the strength of your abdominal muscles to keep the ball moving straight out in front of you, rather than swerving off to the side.

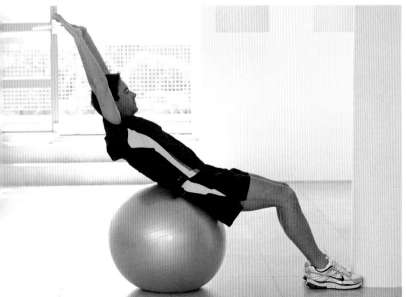

8 swiss ball crunches
(30–60 reps)

Sit on a Swiss ball at a 45° angle. The higher up the ball you sit, the greater the challenge. With arms crossed over your chest, using only your abdominal muscles (not your back muscles), raise your torso and lower it again without going so far as to sit upright or lie horizontally.

Progression: Extend your arms straight above your head, close to your ears (see left). You can also hold a weight or medicine ball above your chest to increase resistance while you crunch upwards.

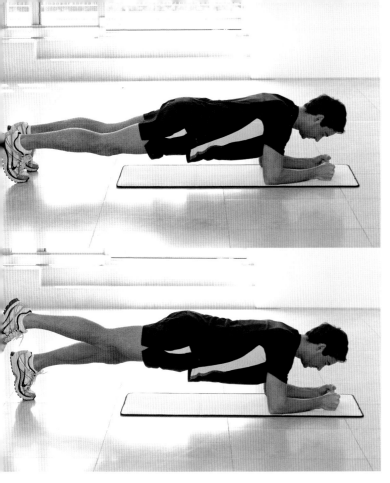

9 plank

(hold for 30–60 secs)

In a push-up position, with forearms flat on the ground, hold your body straight and flat, with glutes and core muscles pulled in tight. Don't allow your pelvis to sag or your bum to stick up in the air.

Progression: Lift each foot off the ground for half the time.

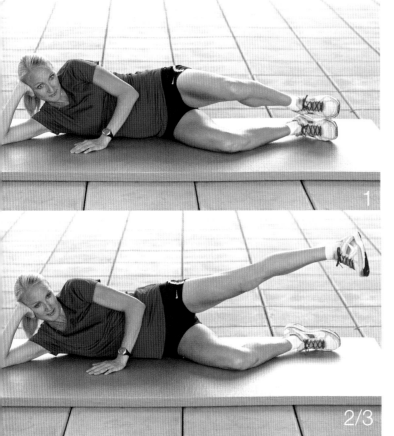

10 mini glute circuit

(30–60 seconds each without pause x 1–2 sets)

Do the following three exercises consecutively without a pause on one side. Repeat for the other side.

1 Lie on your side with your knees drawn up and use your glutes to raise and lower your upper leg.

Progression: Tie an exercise band around your knees to create resistance. Repeat.

2 Straighten your legs and remove the band. Pull your toes towards you, raise your upper leg and take it slightly back behind you (feel your glute working). Gently bounce or do small foot circles.

3 Now move the straight upper leg slightly forward of your pelvis and, keeping toes pulled up, repeat the small foot circles.

2/3

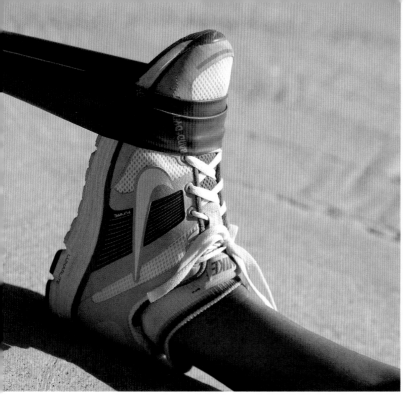

foot strengthening exercises

You'll need to do these at least once a week if you have weak feet and/or shin problems.

peroneal exercises

(10–15 reps each time x 2 sets each side)
You have three peroneus muscles in your lower leg, the longest of which runs under the foot and attaches to the fifth metatarsal. It helps you go up on your toes, as well as pulling the outside of the foot upwards, and it can get very tight, particularly in road-runners.
Try this:
Tie an exercise band around a solid table leg. Lying flat or seated, loop the band around your toes. Pull toes straight back towards you for 10–15 reps. Now turn the foot inwards for 10–15 reps, then outwards.

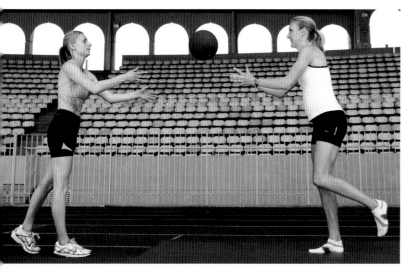

proprioception (balance) exercises

You need only five minutes every couple of days to do these – you can even do them while brushing your teeth, so there's no excuse for not fitting them into your schedule!

single-leg balance

(hold for 60 seconds each side)
Stand without shoes on one leg on a mat or a towel with the knee very slightly bent (locking it out straight is cheating – you won't be gaining much from it).
Progression 1: Do this with your eyes closed.
Progression 2: Try catching and throwing a medicine ball to a partner (with your eyes open!).

single-leg put-down-and-lift

(10–15 reps x 2 sets each side)
Standing on one leg, bend to place a tennis ball or empty cup on the floor, and then bend to pick it up with the other hand. Move round to place it in different positions around you. Repeat for the other side.

sample weights sessions

It's just impossible to be exact about a resistance (weights) programme in a book. The best exercises for you will depend on the equipment available to you and whether or not you have a training partner who can act as a 'spotter'.

A 'spotter' is someone who will help you get the weights into position at the beginning of an exercise and keep a watchful eye on you as you perform it, ready to help if need be. Plus, of course, give you encouragement.

I've come up with three examples of programmes to give you a basic idea, labelled Sessions A, B and C. You'll see references to these sessions when you get to the training programmes later in the book. At that point, turn back to the page listed to find the resistance exercises that are appropriate to your level of experience.

The rules for every session
• Always warm up well to prepare the muscles before you so much as touch a weight – either a short cycle or jog, plus a good stretch.
• Where you see 'warm-up set', perform just one set of the exercise that follows, using light and easy weights.
• Allow a couple of minutes' recovery between sets – you can use down-time to stretch or do a recovery exercise.
• Perform more reps when you're using lighter weights; fewer reps with heavier weights.
Now apply these rules to your weight-training programme.

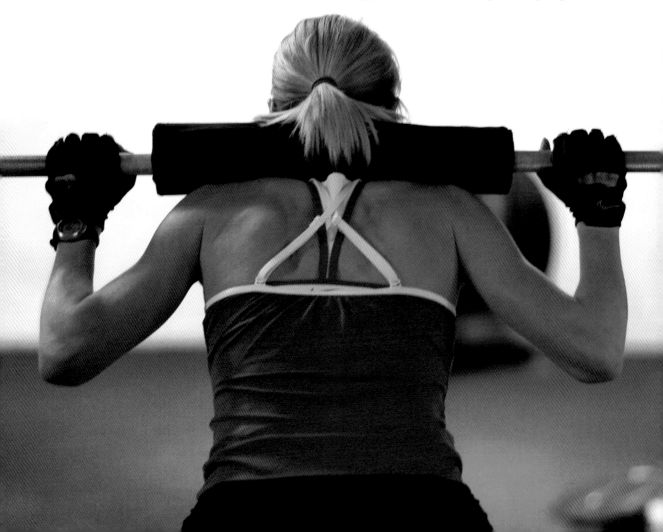

sample session A

Overhead squats
with a light bar
or rod

With shoulders back, hips level and shoulder blades squeezed together, grasp a light bar with a wide grip. Follow instructions for the squat below, bar above your head with elbows straight and arms fully extended, going only as low as you can while holding the position.
Progression: Perform this standing on a wobble board or two Bosu balls.

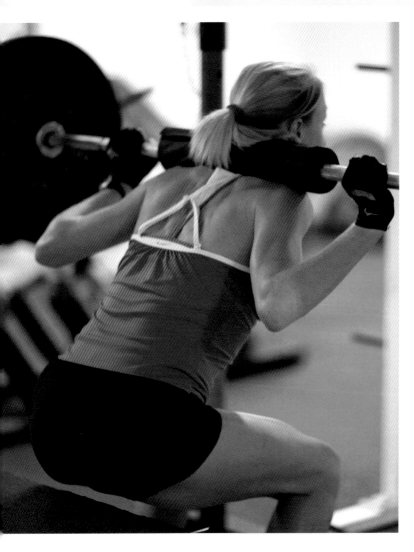

Regular squats or dumbbell squats
(6–10 reps x 3 sets)

This can be done without weights if you're new to weight-training or, more commonly, with a barbell. If you're using dumbbells to add extra resistance, hold them in place on each shoulder. Position your feet slightly wider than hip-width apart and direct your gaze straight in front of you. Bending at the knees, lower your body and push your bum backwards as though you're about to sit down on a chair. Drop to the point where your thighs are as close to parallel to the floor as possible. Concentrate on keeping your hips level, your core strong and your back straight. Extend your bum out behind you. Lower steadily, hold for a second at the bottom, then push back up quickly and explosively.

60-second seated
'running arms'

Sitting on the floor with good posture, legs straight out in front of you, perform a fast forward/backward running action with your arms, concentrating on good arm technique. The momentum you build up should cause your bum to 'walk' slightly forward on the floor during the 60 seconds.

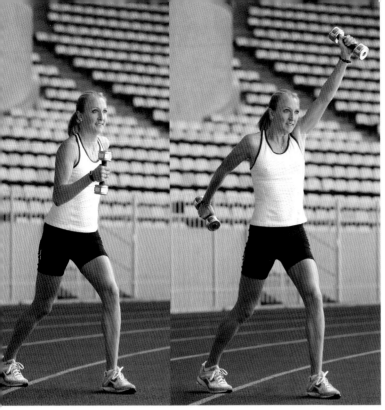

warm-up set

curl to press
(8–10 each side x 2 sets)
Stand with your arms down by your sides and a dumbbell in each hand. Alternately curl the weights up to each shoulder, one at a time, keeping your elbow close to your side; then punch upwards with your arm straight above your head, as you extend the other arm behind you.

hamstring curls on the ball
(10–12 reps x 2 sets)
With shoulders on the floor and heels on the ball, squeeze your glutes and raise your hips to create a straight line from shoulders to feet. Using your heels, roll the ball in towards your bum, then roll it back out again, keeping the hips high.

Progression:
one-leg hamstring curls on the ball
(8–10 reps)
Perform this the same way, but this time with only one leg on the ball.

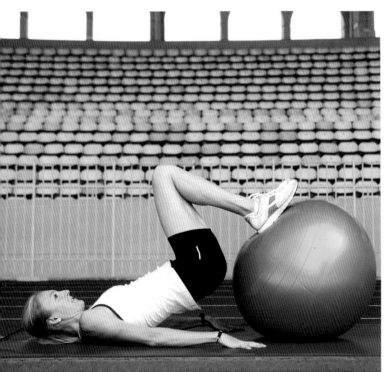

abs circuit
Mix up a variety of abdominal core strength exercises from the 'Core strength training programme' section on pages 49-53 of this chapter (e.g. sets of medicine ball twists, Swiss ball roll-outs, Swiss ball crunches and windscreen wipers).

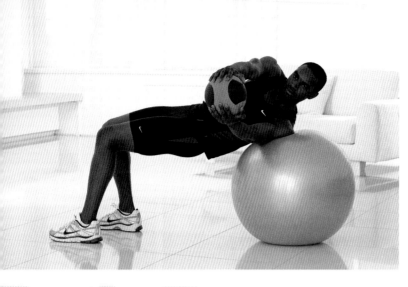

sample session B

warm-up set

Russian twists

(8–10 reps to each side)

Form a bridge with head and shoulders on a Swiss ball, a 90° angle at the knees, glutes squeezed and hips high. Holding a weight above your chest with straight, immobile arms, use only your side muscles (obliques) to twist your upper body first on to one shoulder (on the ball), then the other.

lunges with dumbbells or barbell

(8–10 reps each side x 2–3 sets)

With front and back knees bent to 90°, back knee hovering just above the ground, hold the dumbbells at your side and, with alternate legs, lunge forward and push up and back to the start. Keep your body upright, your back straight and your core and pelvis stable.

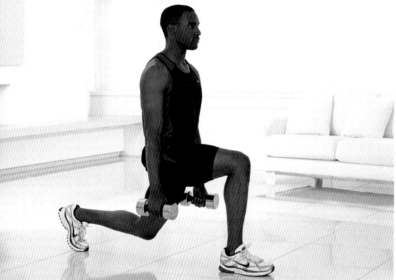

Progression:

single-leg lunge squat

Perform exactly the same movement, but with your back foot on a bench and holding the weights on your shoulders. Do all 8–10 reps on the same leg before switching legs. Don't let your knee travel forward in front of your toes.

optional
recovery exercise

calf raises

During rest intervals between sets, perform 10 double-leg calf raises x 1 set and 10 single-leg calf raises x 2 sets: stand with the balls of both feet on the edge of a stair or low bench, heels hanging off it. Go up on to your toes to full extension and slowly down again. Repeat, doing one leg at a time.

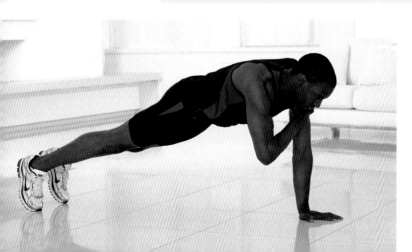

warm-up set

alternate arm tap

(10 reps each side)

In a straight-arm, push-up position, lift each hand off the floor in turn to tap the opposite shoulder. Take great care to keep abs and glutes contracted, as well as bum down and hips level so that your body is in a completely straight line throughout.

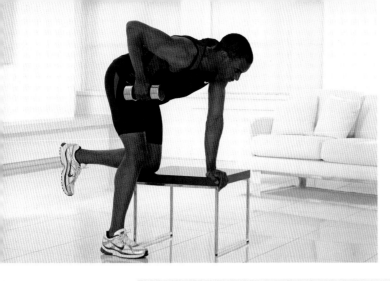

single-arm row
(30–60 secs each without pause x 1–2 sets)
With a dumbbell in your right hand, place your left knee and left arm on the near side of a bench. The right supporting foot is on the floor and knees are aligned. Your back is flat and your navel drawn in towards your spine. Leading with the elbow and keeping it close to your side, raise the dumbbell all the way up to your chest without twisting your torso or hiking up your shoulder blade – your back stays perfectly level throughout.

optional
recovery exercise

assisted pull-ups or lat pull-downs
These two exercises require gym equipment, so if you have membership of a local gym, ask an instructor for help and learn how to perform them with good technique.

4-exercise upper body circuit
(6 reps of each exercise x 2–3 sets)
This can also be used on its own as part of a lighter taper workout (see 'taper exercises' in each of the race distance training programmes), as well as being part of the main workout. Focus on keeping your abs pulled in tightly throughout.

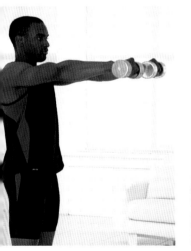 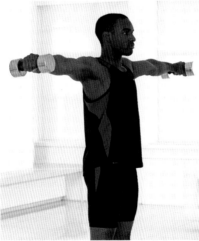 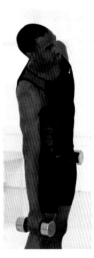 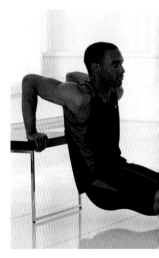

1 front straight-arm raises
With feet shoulder-width apart, dumbbells at your sides, lift them straight ahead to shoulder height, then slowly lower.

2 lateral straight-arm raises
Adopt the same stance, but this time raise the dumbbells out to each side until level with shoulders, then slowly lower.

3 side bends
Same stance, back straight and dumbbells hanging by sides, lower them slowly to the right and left, feeling the stretch.

4 triceps dip off a bench
With straight legs, lower your bum to the floor, then push up to straighten your arms. Keep elbows tucked into sides.

abs circuit

Pick a few abdominal core strength exercises from 'Core strength training programme' on pages 49–53 (e.g. medicine ball twists, Swiss ball roll-outs/crunches, windscreen wipers).

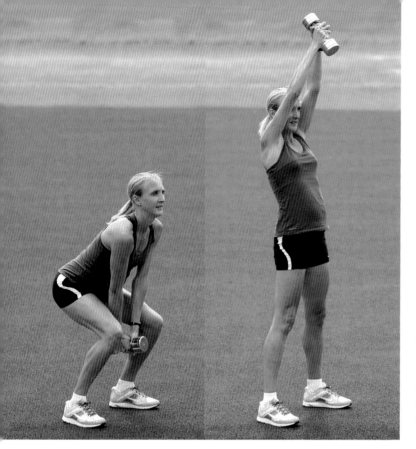

sample session C

These are optional, and only for those following the advanced (sub-elite) runners' programme.

warm-up set

kettle swings
(10 reps x 2 sets)
Standing with feet slightly wider than shoulder-width apart, take one dumbbell in both hands. Keep your back straight, shoulder blades pulled back and gaze directed forwards. Push your pelvis and bum back, bend your knees and drop the dumbbells back between and behind your legs. Drive up with your legs, pushing the pelvis forward and squeezing the glutes hard. Keeping your arms and wrists straight, swing the dumbbell to just above head height.

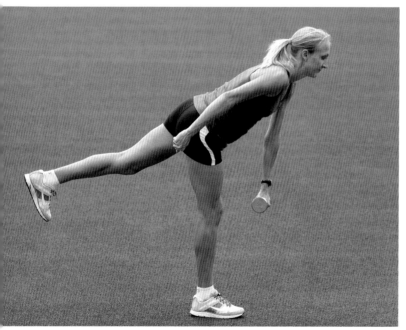

single-leg Russian deadlifts
(8–10 reps x 2)
Stand on one leg with a dumbbell in the opposite hand. Keeping your core muscles strong and shoulders back, your back flat and straight, lower the dumbbell slowly towards the ground while extending the leg you're not standing on straight back behind you. Keep your weight tipped back on to the heel of the supporting foot to maximise the effect on the glutes and hamstrings. Hold for a second at your end range and then straighten back up.

optional
recovery exercise

calf raises
During rest intervals between sets, do 10 double-leg calf raises x 1 set and 10 single-leg calf raises x 2 sets. Stand with the balls of both feet on the edge of a step or stair, heels hanging off it. Go up on to your toes to full extension and slowly down again. Repeat, one leg at a time.

warm-up set

60-second seated 'running arms'

Sitting on the floor with good posture, legs straight out in front of you, perform a fast front-back-front running action with your arms, concentrating on good arm technique. The momentum you build up should cause your bum to 'walk' slightly forward across the floor.

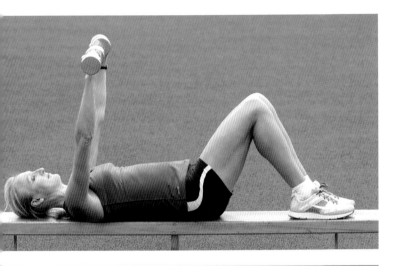

bench press

(6–8 reps x 2-3 sets)

Lie face-up on a bench. Hold dumbbells just above chest with a 90º angle at the elbows. Your elbows are tucked in close to your sides. Lift them directly above your chest, until your arms are nearly fully extended, but the elbows are soft, arcing them in towards each other so that they meet in the middle above your chest. If you're using a barbell, start in the same way, but lift it directly above your chest until your arms are nearly fully extended but the elbows are soft; then lower to the starting position.

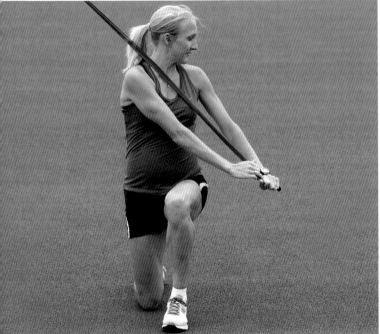

kneeling cable (or exercise band) wood chop

Kneel with your side facing the point at which the cable (or exercise band) is attached, just above head height. With a double-handed grip and tension already on the cable when your arms are stretched upwards, pull your arms down across your body and extend them out to the other side. Concentrate on keeping your glutes and core strong, and feel the effect on your stomach muscles.

abs circuit

Mix up a variety of abdominal core strength exercises from the 'Core strength training programme' section on page 49–53 of this chapter. (e.g. sets of medicine ball twists, Swiss ball roll-outs, Swiss ball crunches and windscreen wipers).

symptoms to look out for...

As I know all too well, you can be perfectly fit and healthy one day only to have something go wrong the next. Whether it's sudden injury or repetitive strain that creeps up over time, the rule is always the same: don't soldier on or you'll risk permanent damage – get it examined and diagnosed.

This needn't necessarily mean that you have to stop training altogether. There's usually something you can be getting on with while an injury is healing. It might be upper body weight training, or strengthening your abdominal muscles, or a different form of cardio such as aqua jogging, bike or cross-trainer that takes the pressure off the injury. Meanwhile, apply the RICE treatment: Rest it, Ice it, Compress it (depending on the nature of the injury) and Elevate it (sit with the afflicted limb up) until you can see a medical professional.

Achilles tendonitis occurs when the tendon at the back of your leg that connects your lower leg muscles to your heel bone becomes inflamed. It has a habit of coming and going so that you sometimes think you're in the clear, then, irritatingly, you become aware that you're not. Head it off by stretching your Achilles tendon after every run (see calf stretch on page 45) and by doing ice cup massage (see 'Top tip' below). If the pain perseveres, get professional attention.
Top tip: Keep empty yoghurt pots or plastic cups of ice in the freezer. At the first sign of soreness, take one out and massage the area for 10–12 minutes. This is more effective than an ice wrap or pack, as you benefit from additional massage action without the danger of ice burns.

Arch pain is inflammation that can have several causes; plantar fasciitis (see opposite page) is one of them (although the pain is more usually felt in the heel). The posterior tibialis tendon also attaches at the arch and when inflamed can cause it to drop painfully. A stress fracture of the bone that supports the arch could also be the culprit. For under-arch pain, always consult a sports medicine specialist and don't run until you've been given the all clear. If it is plantar fascia tightness, rolling the foot on a massage ball/tennis ball can help stretch the muscles.

Athlete's Foot is a fungal infection that thrives in moist, airless conditions and is usually first noticed between the toes. Your running shoes provide the perfect environment. Don't walk barefoot in changing rooms, where it's easily transmitted from foot to foot, and dry properly between your toes. Talk to your local pharmacist about over-the-counter remedies (sprays, creams and powders).

Anaemia or iron depletion is another classic distance runner's problem. Runners are at risk of losing more iron than their sedentary brethren through the heavy sweating and repetitive foot pounding that can cause capillaries to break down and blood cells to rupture. Our bodies are also constantly trying to produce more red blood cells to help us exercise more efficiently – for this we need a good store of iron. The risk for female runners is compounded by menstruation (see Chapter 10). If you feel chronically tired and your fitness levels are dropping despite your best efforts, ask your doctor to measure your serum ferritin – this tests for depleted iron stores. Work to prevent this by eating iron-rich foods combined with vitamin C- and B-rich foods daily. (See Chapter 9, Eat to win.)

Amenorrhea (See Chapter 10, Focus on women.)

Black toenail is a classic sign of running in shoes that are either too big or too small. Toes that continually bump or rub against the toe box can become bruised, and the nail can lift away from the nail bed, causing it to develop a blood blister under the nail. Because there's little air there, it takes longer than normal to heal, hence the somewhat alarming appearance. Head it off by buying correctly fitting shoes (running shoes tend to be half a size bigger than your day shoes – see 'If your shoe fits, wear it', page 20); making sure your socks are suitable (see 'Socks are important, too', page 24); and keeping your toenails short.

Blisters are the result of chafing (see opposite page). Place a prophylactic over it – this acts as a second skin, cushioning it and keeping it bacteria-free while it heals. When you're breaking in new shoes, apply one at the first sign of rubbing. If, however, you have sweaty feet like me, a prophylactic won't work. The danger is that it can come unstuck as you run, wrinkling and causing further painful blisters. I apply anti-chafing cream to my feet before long runs and races to prevent blisters. If I'm unfortunate enough to develop any, I paint the area with a varnish specifically designed for this purpose and allow it to dry. Ask your local pharmacist for advice on the best brands for this purpose.

Chafing is caused by repeated rubbing of skin against skin or skin against fabric, the latter usually due to ill-fitting clothing. Trouble spots lie around the bra line, inner thighs, under-arms and, for men, the nipple area. Sweat worsens the abrasive effect. If you run in clothing specifically designed for running, you shouldn't have this problem.

Applying an anti-chafing cream to vulnerable spots before short runs can help, but long runs need a more permanent solution. The synthetic fabric of running-specific technical clothing wicks moisture away and has flattened seams that sit softly against the skin. (Cotton is the worst offender: over a long run its roughness turns it into a scourer – once wet it can rub skin raw.) Gentlemen, the time-honoured practice of sticking-plasters placed over nipples does help prevent chafing.

Cramps can have a few origins: dehydration is the No. 1 culprit – not just while you're out running, but inadequate fluid intake in the hours beforehand can be enough to do the damage. If you're doing big mileage in hot weather, you might find that cramps, combined with a feeling of muscle weakness, benefit from a little additional salt – with strong emphasis on the word 'little'. Potassium depletion is another possible cause: we know that when the body needs more of this electrolyte it can trigger a muscle spasm, a.k.a. cramp; so make a point of upping your intake of potassium-rich foods, such as bananas, squash, spinach, avocado, oranges, tomatoes, potatoes and sweet potatoes, prunes and raisins. Increasing muscle strength and suppleness can also help.

Hamstring pulls are small tears in the muscles at the back of the thighs. They are more commonly associated with sprinting than distance running, but sudden acceleration under any circumstances can be the culprit. Rest and ice are the immediate treatment – if there's no improvement, get medical attention.

Plantar fasciitis is a common complaint among runners, because running big mileages can stress the heel bone. This painful heel condition happens when the plantar fascia (the tough band of tissue that supports the bottom of your foot and connects your heel bone to your toes) becomes inflamed. There can be several reasons:

inflexibility of the calf muscles, lack of arch support (see an expert about possible orthotic inserts), wearing running shoes that are well past their throw-out date, carrying too much weight and suddenly (rather than gradually) increasing physical activity. Sometimes the problem can be something biomechanical that's peculiar to you. If it persists, see a sports physiotherapist, but in the first instance, rest your feet, ice them and stretch them by rolling the foot on a tennis ball or massage ball.

Iliotibial Band Syndrome (ITBS) The iliotibial band runs from the hip to just below the knee on the outer side of the shinbone. It works with the thigh muscles in a gliding action; this allows the knee to bend while also keeping it stable. When it becomes inflamed, the gliding movement becomes painful and less fluent. Causes can be increased mileage, overpronation, or sometimes worn-out running shoes. Give it immediate rest, ice it and seek professional help. Foam roller massage can really help here.

Shin splints are an inflammation of the tendon on the outer edge of the tibia (the bone at the front of the lower leg). It is most often associated with muscle over-use, or over-training, and the impact of repeated landings on hard surfaces. Check that your shoes aren't past their throw-out date and that they are correct for your gait. When you're ready to train again, start on grass while your body re-adjusts. It is useful to have a biomechanist look at your gait to make sure there aren't any biomechanical problems that need to be sorted out, and to prescribe special stretches. Meanwhile, rest, ice your shins and try to sit with your leg/legs up as much as possible. Massaging up and down the shins with an ice cup can help.

Stress fractures are small cracks in bone, usually ascribed to doing too much, too soon, too quickly. One of running's great benefits is that the impact causes the body to create bone, which increases its density. We lay down new bone and take away old bone in a smooth cycle. However, runners who sharply increase their training in too short a time period are asking the body to work too quickly and the cycle gets out of sync. The initial result is bony oedema, a first sign on scans that the bone is under stress. If the stress is allowed to continue, a fracture line will appear, signalling a full-blown stress fracture. The only treatment is rest from impact and no running until a bony callus forms and hardens over the crack. Ask a sports physiotherapist about alternative, non-weight-bearing cardio exercise to keep your fitness levels up while you heal. Also, be sure your diet contains enough calcium and vitamin D.

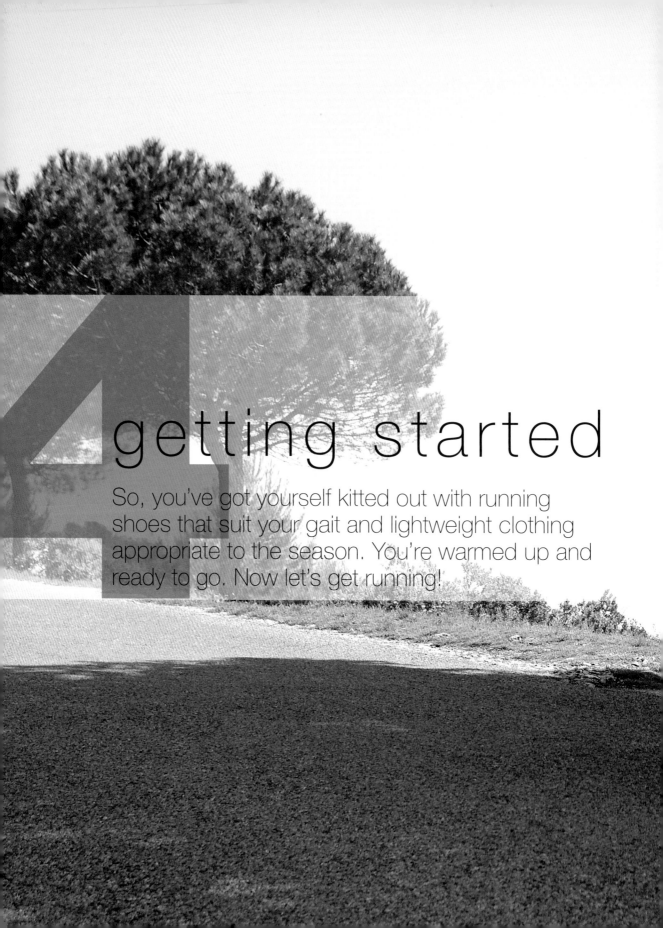

4 getting started

So, you've got yourself kitted out with running shoes that suit your gait and lightweight clothing appropriate to the season. You're warmed up and ready to go. Now let's get running!

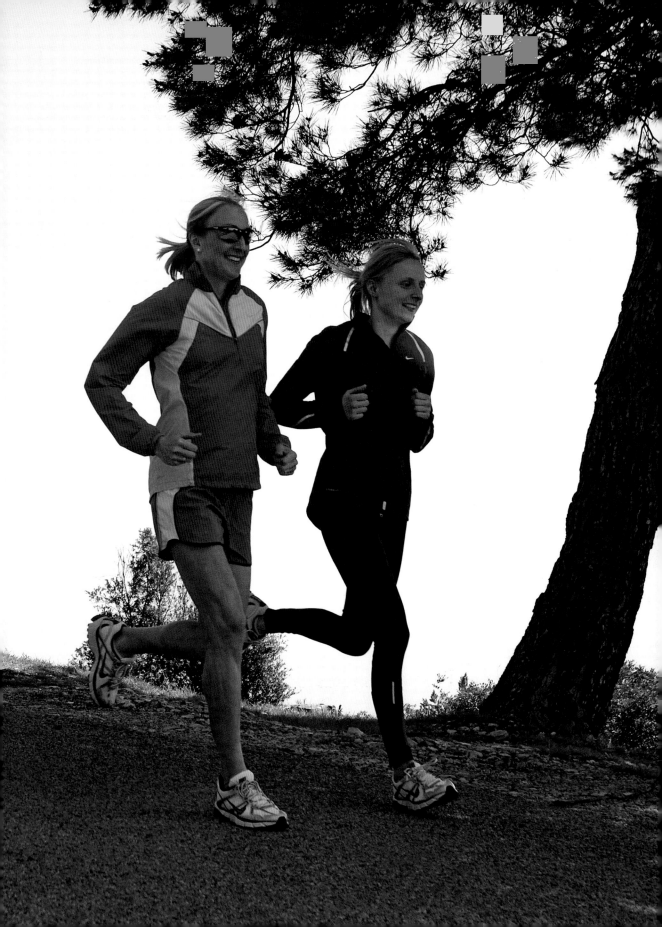

run with friends

One of the easiest ways to get more out of your running is to join a group or club. It introduces you to a whole new circle of friends and opens up another window on your social life.

Mutual encouragement is the payoff that comes from being part of a group – it does wonders for helping keep you motivated when you feel yourself flagging. Rarely will all of you be feeling tired or having a hard day at the same time; this is fortunate, as there will be occasions when you'll be relying on your running mates to help pull you through a bad patch. It also makes you look forward to your runs and ensures that you turn up for them on time. In practical terms, too, there's safety in numbers.

Look for a running club in your area. Most of them cater for all-comers, with groups built around different ability levels. This is useful when you're getting started, as your new running friends will include people who are more experienced than you and can help you out by answering queries and offering advice.

However, it doesn't have to be a club. Just getting together with a group of friends once a week can enhance your running experience. A good way is to link up informally with people whose goal is to use a particular race as a means of raising money for a charity. You'll then have an even greater – and higher – motive for sticking at it.

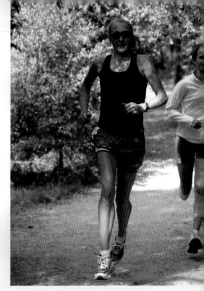

running club

- Do a Google search for clubs in your area, or phone your local Council's Sport & Recreation Department.
- Ask them these questions:
  - Is there a qualified coach to advise on training?
  - How many organised training runs are there per week and what type (time trials, long runs, etc)?
  - Are there membership benefits (discounts on kit, race entry fees, and so on)?

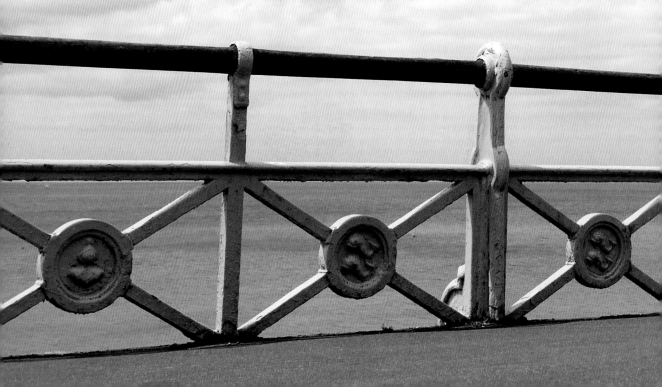

'There will be occasions when you'll be relying on your running mates to help pull you through a bad patch'

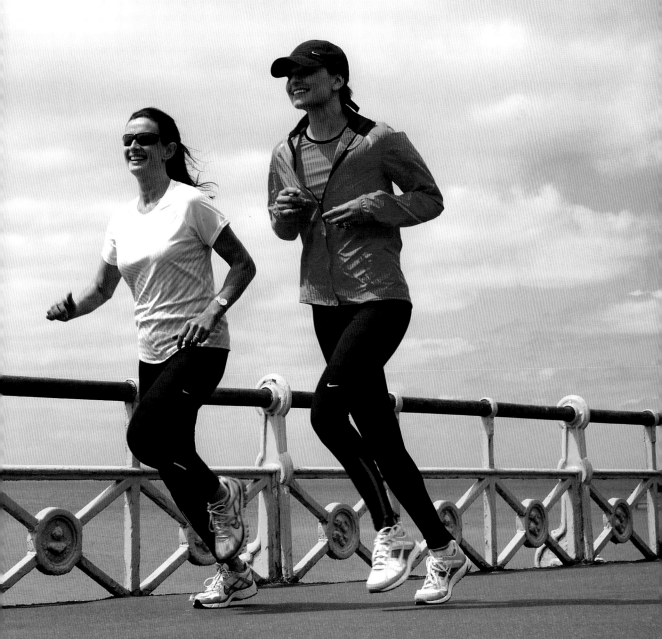

chart your progress

Once you've written out your reasons for running and your goals (see Chapter 1, Set your goals) you're good to go. However, one thing I recommend is that you pick a method of recording and charting your running that shows your progress over time.

This can be as simple as noting your training results on a calendar or wall planner as you go along, or keeping a dedicated online diary or a pocket-book version. If you opt for a diary, I find the best layout is week-to-view, as it gives you enough space to fit in everything you need to record each day and allows you to look back over a week without having to flip between pages.

For each training session, write down exactly what you did as regards times and distances. This can be as detailed or as simple as you like. For example: lap of the park in 22 minutes or five-mile progression with mile splits ('splits' is the term for the time taken to run each mile, e.g. 10 mins, 9.53, 9.50, 9.47, 9.46). Make a note of the weather conditions, too, especially if there were extremes of

january	monday	tuesday	wednesday
resting heart rate			
weight			
time of day of run			
weather conditions			
distance run/ duration of run			
mile splits (time per mile)			
how I felt			

temperature or it was windy. You'll need to be able to look back, compare sessions and identify any variable that may have affected your times on certain days. I also add how I felt during the run. For example: good, tired or sluggish setting off; tired during; or legs feeling good or achy. If I used a heart rate monitor on a run (see Chapter 5, Raising your game, for more about monitors) I write down my average and maximum heart rates for the session. It's important to log any aches and pains, ankle twists and so on, however minor, so that you can refer to them later should problems develop. Chart what you do on non-running days, too, as this can affect how you feel the next day – especially if you spent a whole day shopping, did a long car journey, or had a night out.

Stress will also affect how you feel. Having said that, aerobic activity is renowned as one of the all-time great stress relievers. A training run or, indeed, any aerobic activity such as circuit training or body pump, can generate up to two hours of what's called 'post-exercise euphoria'. This is also known as the 'endorphin response'. Endorphins are the feel-good neurotransmitters released by the brain when you exercise. They improve your mood and leave you in a more relaxed state. Think of how terrific you feel after you've finished a run or a workout, even if the session was hard work while you were actually doing it. What's more, it's uninterrupted time in which you're left to your own wandering thoughts or your favourite music. Plus, you can choose a beautiful, natural environment in which to run that will expunge all traces of work from your mind. My best thinking time is while I'm out running. Maybe it's due to increased oxygen to the brain, but my problems become clearer and my world seems more settled and ordered by the time I get back. The appeal of running is a no-brainer, right?

thursday	friday	saturday	sunday

lose a few pounds?

If one of your goals is to lose weight, then choose a day to weigh yourself, stick to the same time on the same day every week, wear exactly the same clothes, and record it in your diary.

However, don't fall into the trap of doing this any more frequently, as it can spiral into an unhealthy obsession with the scales. Your weight varies as the day progresses and, for women, with the hormonal fluctuations of the menstrual cycle. Not only that, but scales give only half the picture, anyway. Muscle weighs more than fat, so once your body starts to tone and shape up, the scales may not show much progress, even if you do!

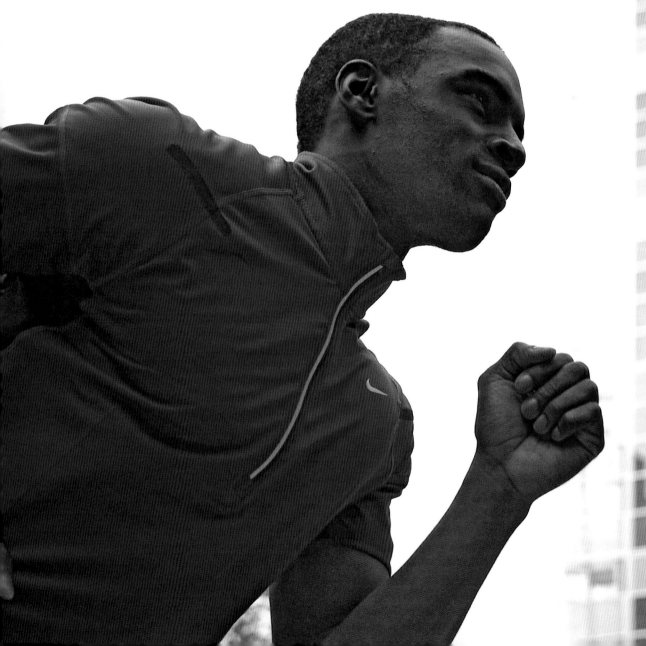

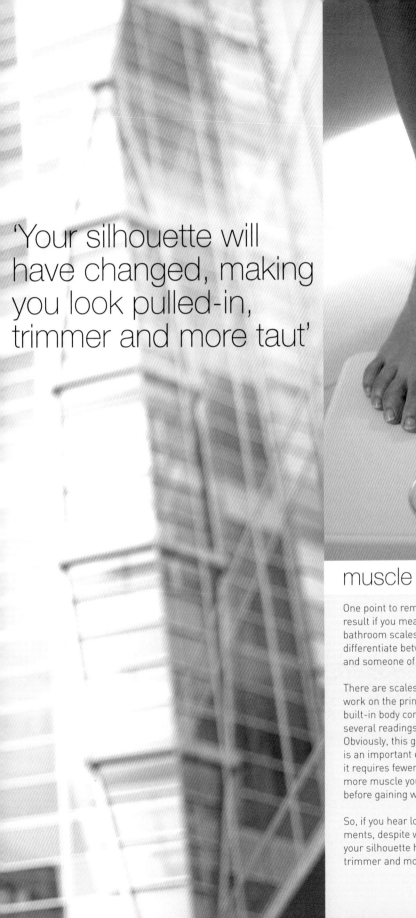

'Your silhouette will have changed, making you look pulled-in, trimmer and more taut'

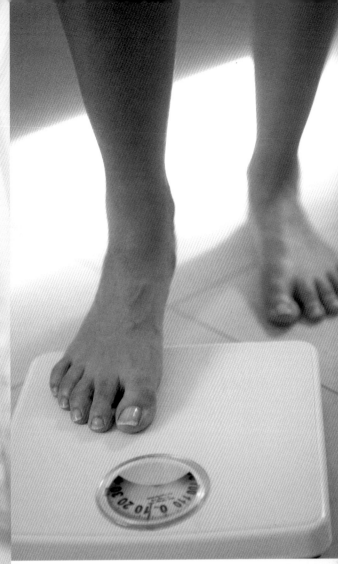

muscle weighs more than fat

One point to remember is that you get a more accurate result if you measure your body composition. Standard bathroom scales give your total weight, but they can't differentiate between a 70kg, well-muscled individual and someone of the same weight who is simply fat.

There are scales on the market that can do this; they work on the principle of bioelectrical impedance – a built-in body composition measurement that can give several readings, including body fat and muscle mass. Obviously, this gives you a much truer picture. Body fat is an important element in successful weight control – it requires fewer calories than muscle, so the less fat/more muscle you have, the more calories you can eat before gaining weight.

So, if you hear lots of 'Wow, you've lost weight' comments, despite what the scales tell you, it's because your silhouette has changed, making you look pulled-in, trimmer and more taut.

monitor your heart rate

Another important item to record, especially if you're doing a fair amount of training, is your resting heart rate. Take it in the morning before you move – even sitting up in bed will elevate it slightly, so measure it while you're still recumbent and relaxed.

HOW TO MEASURE YOUR RESTING HEART RATE

Before you go to sleep, put a clock that has a second hand, or has the seconds clearly visible, on the bedside table where you can see it without having to make any more of an effort than turning your head. If you forget and sit up in bed, abandon the attempt and do it the following day. Locate your pulse in advance – I find it's easiest to place the tips of my fingers on the top of my neck, just below the jawbone – either side of the neck works equally well. (Don't use your thumb, because it has a pulse of its own, which could be confusing.) You're now pressing down just over your carotid artery, which will give you a more

obvious beat than your wrist. However, if you do happen to be able to feel it strongly at your wrist, this works just the same.

Either count the number of beats over 60 seconds, or just count the number of heart beats over 10 seconds and multiply the figure by 6 to give you the number of beats per minute (bpm). This is a good indicator: the fitter you become, the lower your resting heart rate. More importantly, an increased morning pulse can be a valuable sign of either over-training or incipient illness. If it's up a few beats, give yourself one or two easy days; however, if it rises significantly (five beats or more) take a couple of days

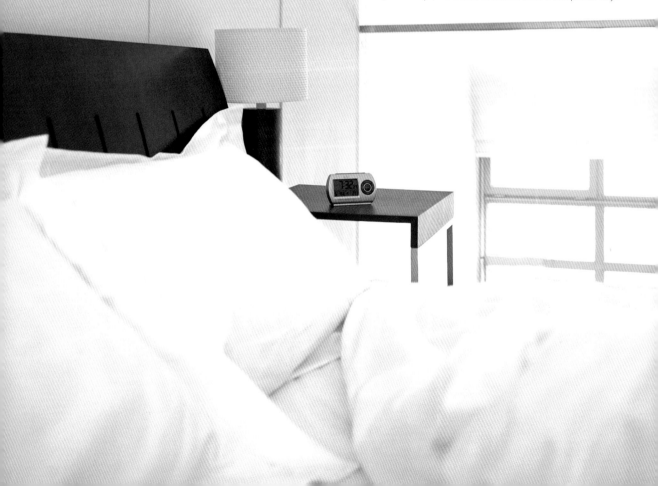

off until it returns to normal. I've avoided succumbing to a full-blown cold or virus on several occasions by heeding this handy warning sign. Make a note of your resting heart rate in your training diary every time you take it.

The value in keeping a diary is that it enables you to observe how your running is going day to day, and whether it's improving over time. As the data accumulates, it becomes a valuable training aid. If you have a very good run or race, you can easily look back and pick out the training that worked for you. Conversely, if you feel tired or stale, you might look back and see that your training has been too similar recently, or that it has been a long time since you last took a break. It might also just be that your child's chickenpox, or first attempts to go through nights without nappies, affected you more than you had thought. Or perhaps it's just that you always feel tired after the indulgence of Christmas and New Year.

Generally speaking, if you train regularly you'll usually find that you have a lower resting heart rate than many of your sedentary friends and colleagues. This is because exercise trains the heart to pump more blood (and hence, oxygen) round the body with each beat. As a very rough guide, under 70 is good, below 60 is very good, and below 50 is pretty impressive.

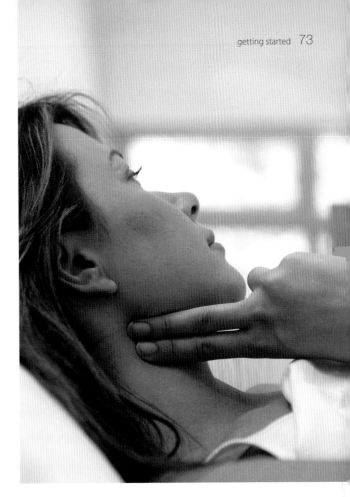

alternative way to check your pulse

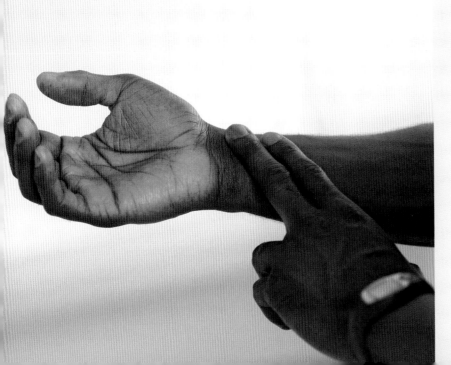

use your wrist

- Place the pads of the index finger and middle finger of one hand on the inside of your opposite wrist, in line with the base of your thumb.
- If, at first, it's difficult to detect any heartbeat at all, press down more firmly and move your fingers around until you find it.
- Monitor its rhythm for half a minute or so to make sure it's regular, then count the number of beats for 10 seconds. Mutiply this figure by six, and you'll have your resting heart rate/pulse.

build up gradually

If you're new to running, you'll derive a lot of motivation and satisfaction from picking a goal of, say, a 5K Race For Life. Choose one that's due to take place in two to three months' time (it takes around eight weeks to prepare for a 5K run from scratch).

I always recommend a 5K race as a good initial target to aim for: it's the best possible spur to action you could have, because it conforms perfectly with the requirements of what's known as a 'S.M.A.R.T' goal. This acronym stands for Specific, Measurable, Achievable, Realistic and Timely. Consider how a 5K race matches up: it's very specific (run 5K by a specific date); it's obviously measurable, as there's a detailed training programme against which to benchmark yourself right up to race day; it's highly achievable, in that it's easily accomplished with a bit of training, so this means that it's realistic; plus, with the race as a deadline, there's a definite time frame. The beauty of a S.M.A.R.T. goal is that gives you a very clear focus and a direction around which you can build a schedule. You won't have to guess what you're doing on a particular training day, because you'll already have planned it well ahead of time.

Visit **www.raceforlife.org** and you'll find a race near you on a date that suits.

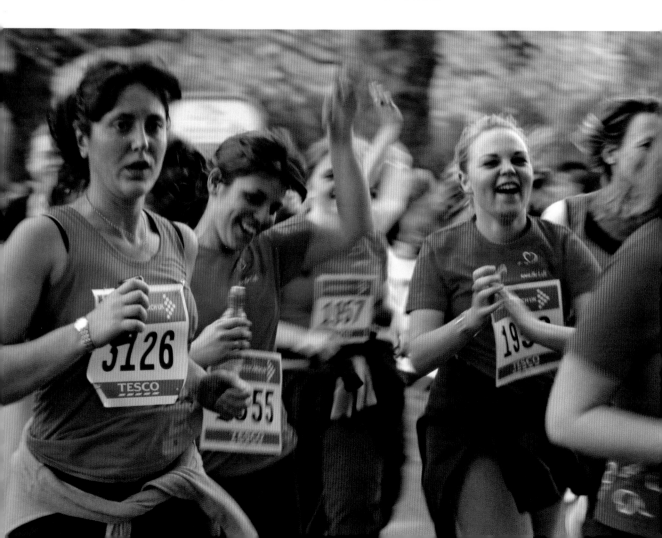

EASY DOES IT

Initially, you'll be focused on building up your fitness levels, but you'll very quickly get beyond that and fall in love with running. In fact, I'd go so far as to say (and this isn't just me saying so – I hear it from runners of all levels everywhere) you'll reach the point where you don't feel right if you don't get your runs in as you want to during the course of a week.

'You'll reach the point where you don't feel right if you don't get your runs in as you want'

Take a few minutes to warm up with gentle jogging before you start (see Chapter 3, Taking care of your body, page 37). Start by alternating short running intervals with short walking intervals; take it slowly and gradually, never adding more than 10% each week. I know people who began their running careers by walking from one lamppost to the next, then running to the next one, and so on, alternately running and walking for 30 minutes. Gradually they worked up to running two lampposts in one go and walking one, then running three lampposts and walking one, then four, and so on until they had joined up all the lampposts and were running continuously. How many minutes you choose to run and then walk is down to your fitness levels when you start off. If you've been a gym-goer for years, or a swimmer or a cyclist, you'll be starting from a base level of greater fitness than someone who might be carrying extra weight, or is older, or coming back from a long period of injury. But resist the urge to increase your mileage suddenly. While you may see your aerobic fitness improve rapidly, your muscles, joints and tendons need time to catch up. Distance running is all about steady, progressive and incremental increases in training.

Lastly, as you'll have read in Chapter 3, after your run don't just stop abruptly – jog, then walk for a few minutes until your breathing is more or less back to normal; then stretch thoroughly before heading for home (read more about stretching on page 42).

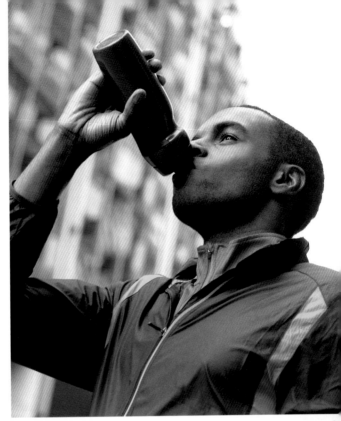

hydration

Make sure you hydrate adequately, particularly in hot weather. Having said that, drinking a load of liquid just before you run could be counter-productive – you may feel bloated and have to run to the sound of sloshing until it's absorbed. Sipping little and often is the key. Start drinking two hours before your run; a couple of glasses of water should do initially, but learn to listen to your body and judge how thirsty you are (read more about the thirst reflex in Chapter 9, Eat to win).

Carry on sipping, and have a last glass or two of water about 20 minutes before you go off on your run. Remember that caffeinated drinks (and, need I say, alcohol!) can have a dehydrating effect and will certainly pass through your body faster, so give them wide berth. Unless it's very hot or you are running for over an hour, you don't need to carry a drink with you. So long as you start well hydrated, you will be fine during your run.

Carrying the bottle, however small, will alter your gait and make running feel more awkward. If you are travelling to training, in the gym, or doing repetition/interval sessions, then take a drink bottle with you and sip little and often. It's a fine – and individual – balance between too much and not enough, but you'll get this right with practice.

age is no barrier!

Never before has so much been written about the benefits of exercise as we age. But then, never before has such a big percentage of the population been heading for the 'third age' all at once.

Thanks to the post-war baby boomers born between 1946 and 1964, everyone is gaining from the research being carried out to prepare society for this demographic tidal wave. One thing is certain, we all need to know how to age well – everyone is on the same journey, only some are a bit further along it than others.

The benefits of acquiring new skills such as languages, crafts and computer know-how, and doing brainteasers like crossword puzzles and Sudoko, have long been known. But it's only now that scientists have begun to

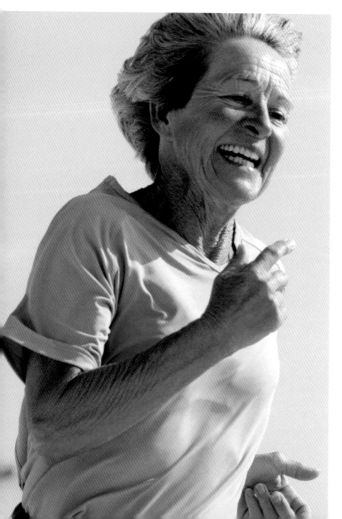

understand the importance of physical exercise to the health of the brain. Until fairly recently, brain deterioration was thought to be an inevitable part of the gradual decline that accompanies ageing. However, many studies reveal that it's quite the opposite: research findings in Cambridge, UK, suggest that new neurons created after exercise can play a role in improving cognitive function. In addition to this, the cardiovascular nature of running raises our heart rate, which in turn exercises the heart muscle. Plus, it maintains the strength of the rest of our musculature: we know that between the ages of 35 and 75 we lose 30% of our muscle mass unless we use it. In fact, much of the so-called age-related decline is shown to be not due to ageing alone, but inactivity. So, lose it or use it!

Having said that, make sure you train and don't strain. In later life, joints are stiffer and muscles take longer to warm up, so heed this advice:

- If you are taking up running in your middle years, get a thorough screening from your doctor first.
- Improve your diet by adding nutrients where lacking (see Chapter 9). There is a view that, as we age, our thirst mechanism becomes dulled and the message doesn't get through as effectively. So keep your fluid levels up.
- Reduce the risk of injury by stretching thoroughly as part of your warm-up and cool-down.
- Limit the quantity and improve the quality of your training: cut back to four days of quality training a week. If you feel short-changed by not doing more, then do some easy, non-load-bearing activity on one of the other days – swimming and cycling are good. One useful tip for older runners that I recently came across is to measure training volume in minutes, not mileage.
- Take at least two full days off per week to recover. From middle age onwards, it's all about training smarter, not harder. Anything other than this tends to lead to injury. If you do a hard training run, for example, take your pulse the following morning: if it's high, you've probably not fully recovered, so be sensible and act accordingly.
- As always, listen to your body!

rest days are important

Initially, it may be hard to think this way about taking time off, but once you're off and loving it, you may find it difficult not to run every day. Rest days can feel as though there's something missing. Forget this thought right now: rest days are a vitally important and integral part of training.

I know it sounds counter-intuitive, but it's in the period after you've trained that your body makes the adaptations necessary to meet the new challenges of training. For weight-lifters, for instance, it's during the days off in between lifting sessions that their muscles repair and build (which is why I said on page 48 that you should only weight-train every other day – never on consecutive days). Endurance training is similar. While for some elite athletes, rest days are for doing light training, most runners factor in time for total rest. In my hard training programme I have a rest day every eight days. I look forward to this on the tough days, plan to do things with my family and

friends that I can't fit in at other times, and find that it refreshes and renews my body and mind for the hard training week ahead. For beginners, rest days mean not doing any running at all. Don't be tempted to ignore this: your body has to adapt gradually to be able to perform to expectation; this means repairing itself, building and strengthening muscles, improving the efficiency of certain chemical functions and increasing lung capacity. If you hammer it with non-stop consecutive training sessions, you'll be leaving no time for recovery, which means no time to develop and get stronger. This can only end in tears, so my advice is: stick with the programme!

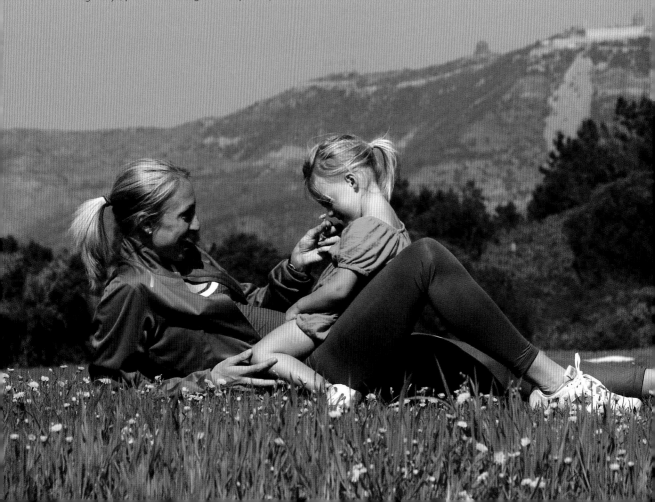

your 5K training programme

Training programmes for beginners can be expressed either in terms of the distance you've run, or the time in which you've completed your run. It's a matter of personal preference, but I always feel it's easier to start off by thinking in terms of the time you've spent running. This saves you the hassle of having to drive around measuring how many blocks make one mile, and so on. Here, for this eight-week training programme example, I've broken it down by time (eight weeks is roughly how long you'll need to prepare for a 5K race). I've assumed that you can already walk a distance of 5K (or 3.1 miles, which is 5,280 yards, if you prefer!) and I've based it on three runs per week at an average running speed of 13 minutes per mile. Don't give up the first time you try following this programme – if it feels a bit like hard work initially, take heart: your fitness levels will pick up, that I promise!

	monday	tuesday	wednesday
week 1	Rest	3-min run/1-min walk 7 repetitions = 28 mins	Rest
week 2	Rest	5-min run/1-min walk 5 reps = 30 mins	Rest
week 3	Rest	7-min run/1-min walk 5 reps = 40 mins	Rest
week 4	Rest	10-min run/1-min walk 4 reps = 44 mins	Rest
week 5	Rest	15-min run/2-min walk 3 reps = 51 mins	Rest
week 6	Rest	25-min run (no walking) 1.9 miles	Rest
week 7	Rest	35-min run (no walking) 2.7 miles	Rest
week 8	Rest	Race week: run for 25 mins (ease off to be strong on race day)	Rest

notes

- I've assumed that the long run will be done by most people on the weekends; but if it suits you to do it on a different day, by all means just schedule the rest of your week's runs around it.

- 'Cross-train' means an easy session of non-running aerobic exercise, e.g. swimming or cycling.

- This programme assumes a speed of 13 mins per mile: bear in mind that it's just a guide – some runners are faster than others.

- As in all things to do with exercise, listen to your body. Learn to watch out for signs of excessive fatigue (rather than an excuse for a lie-in) or viruses, and adjust your programme or take a day's rest accordingly.

thursday	friday	saturday	sunday
Same as Tuesday	Rest	Cross-train	4-min run/1-min walk 6 reps = 30 mins
Same as Tuesday	Rest	Cross-train	6-min run/1-min walk 5 reps = 35 mins
Same as Tuesday	Rest	Cross-train	9-min run/1-min walk 4 reps = 40 mins
Same as Tuesday	Rest	Cross-train	12-min run/1-min walk 4 reps = 52 mins
Same as Tuesday	Rest	Cross-train	20-min run/2-min walk 2 reps = 44 mins
Same as Tuesday	Rest	Cross-train	30-min run (no walking) 2.3 miles
Same as Tuesday	Rest	Cross-train	40-min run (no walking) 3.1 miles (well done!)
Same as Tuesday	Rest	Cross-train	**RACE DAY!**

raising your game

Ready to move on from beginner to intermediate runner? All you need are some technical changes to your training that will improve your performance.

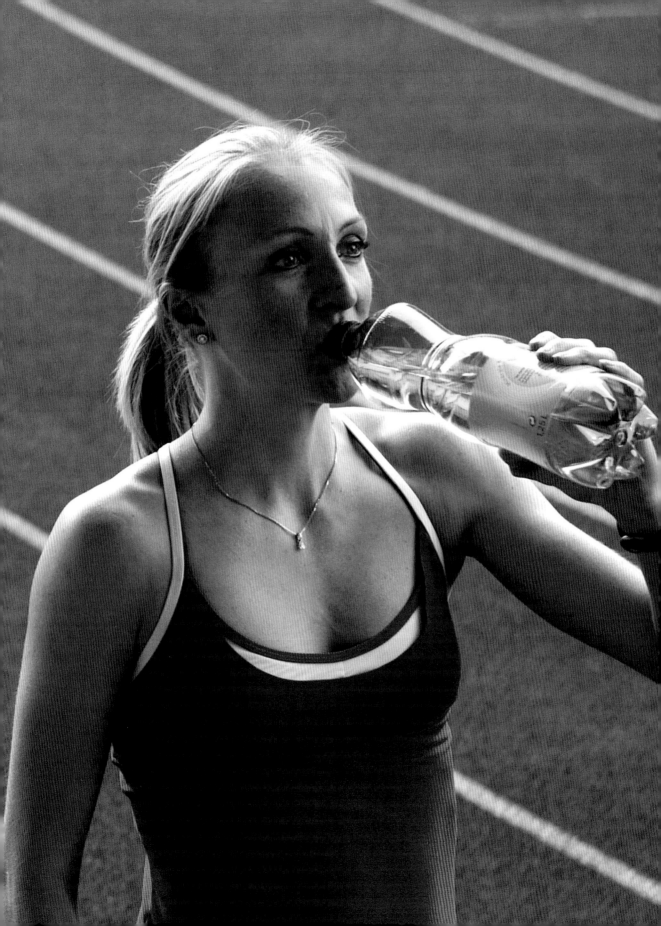

becoming more experienced

I once read an article in *Runner's World* that described the different race distances as follows: 'The 5K is friendly, the 10K is classic, and the half-marathon is a self-esteem-pumping, long-distance race'. To me, that sums it up brilliantly.

In the previous chapter, we discussed how to go about getting started. But what if you've already been there, done that and now want to increase your distances, give yourself a bigger challenge and maybe improve your times? If you're what I call a 'new intermediate', in other words, ready to move up from the 5K beginners' group, you may be thinking about training for a 10K. Of course, you may have already passed this point and have started to step up your mileage, regularly running, say, 20–30 miles a week. In this case, you might be thinking about training for a half-marathon – or even the ultimate challenge of the marathon.

On the other hand, if you're an 'experienced intermediate' who has done these distances a few times and now wants to run them faster, you'll be thinking about what you can do to change and improve your training methods to achieve your goal.

If either of these descriptions fits you, then this chapter may hold some useful tips.

For all runners, good hydration will be an issue on runs of more than 90 minutes. In hot weather, or on longer runs, plan your water stops: parks often provide drinking fountains, so include these in your route, if possible; or ask friends or family to meet you with water at pre-determined points (do this a few times to get in some practice at drinking on the move). Sometimes, on long runs, I even loop around to pass the car or the house every 20–30 minutes so as to practise drink stops. For runs of less than 90 minutes, dehydration should not become an issue as long as you start off well hydrated and rehydrate as soon as you finish your run.

Of course, some people sweat more than others and may need to rehydrate more often. Conversely, the opposite problem sometimes occurs among mass runners in major marathons: hyponatremia. This is massive over-hydration, which leads to very serious health and circulation issues. A good guide in hot weather is to weigh yourself immediately before and after a run. A weight loss of 2% or more will lead to a drop in blood volume, dizziness and, as you'd expect, an impaired performance. If you are losing 2% of your bodyweight over the course of a short run, you really need to hydrate more often.

Another test you should do regulary is the urine check: your urine should preferably be clear, and certainly no darker than the pale lemon colour of straw. Of course, it will be a bit more concentrated after a long run, but it should never be dark or smell strongly. As a last resort, if you can't get a drink along the way, then take an easy-grip, purpose-built water bottle. I say 'last resort' only because gripping anything while you're running is at best an annoyance and at worst could affect your posture and the way you run. Besides, even small irritations can become big ones over long distances.

Runners who sweat a lot will need to pay special attention to their hydration levels. Rather than leave it to guesswork, calculate in advance how much water you lose and from this how much you need to replace when you run. Weigh yourself without your clothes on before a training run and again without them on afterwards. As a rule of thumb, 1lb (500g) of lost body weight equates to 1pint (500ml) of lost water. Divide the duration (counted in minutes) of your run by the amount of water you've lost as a rough guide to how often and by how much you need to top up during your runs.

In racing and in marathon training involving intense running sessions of an hour or longer, it's advisable to think about carbohydrate drinks. As well as containing good electrolyte levels for hydration, these drinks also provide energy. I have a 500ml bottle 2–3 hours before an event and another in the hour before the start. Then during the race I'll take 100–250ml every 5km, depending on weather conditions.

We know pretty conclusively from years of research into sports nutrition that the earlier you refuel after you've finished training, the more quickly your muscles will recover. There's a window of approximately 30 minutes following a hard training session or race during which the muscle cells are at their most receptive to being rebuilt. So, consume at least another 500ml of a recovery drink that will provide a balance of protein and carbohydrate as soon as possible in order to speed muscle recovery and replace the glycogen that you've used up during your session. (Liquid form is preferable to solids, as it's more easily absorbed by the body.)

With greater distances comes an even greater need to pay attention to what you wear. Crucially, shoes must be correctly fitted to suit your gait; seams must not chafe; and clothing needs to be layered so that you can cater for changes in body temperature and weather conditions that may occur over a long run. Have another look at Chapter 2, Getting ready, to make sure you've got all of these essentials covered.

With your footwear and clothing sorted, it's down to making sure that your training programme is a thorough preparation for the distances you want to race, that you stay injury-free and, most of all, that you enjoy yourself.

Don't be scared of longer distances. Almost anyone can do them if they've trained for them and, besides, they're a lot of fun. How else would you get 35,000 people of all ages, shapes and sizes coming from every corner of the globe to participate in the London Marathon? Even more impressive is the fact that not every participant is necessarily in tip-top health: consider how many recovering cancer patients successfully take on this challenge in order to raise money for the charity that has shown them so much support.

This is where the power of the mind and motivation come into play. Determination and steady application can help us all achieve our goals. So, time to get started!

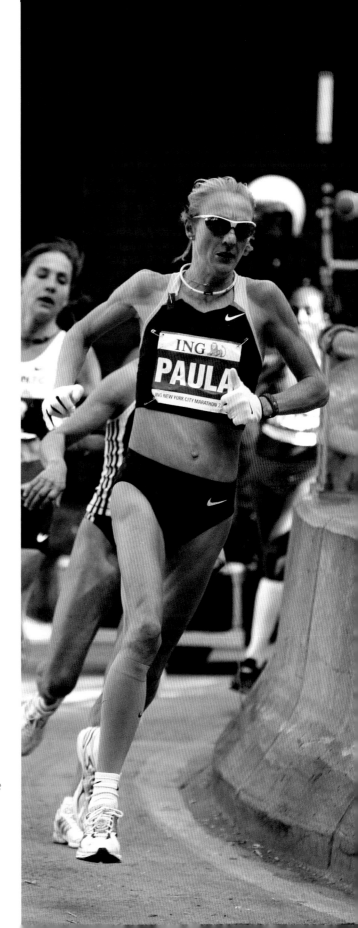

'new intermediate' runners

HOW TO TRAIN FOR A 10K

By this stage, you'll probably be doing a minimum of 10–15 miles over three or four days a week. This might involve running with a training partner, an informal social group, or a club. If the latter, then at least there will be other club members who are well accustomed to doing 10Ks and half-marathons. Seasoned distance runners are usually generous when it comes to sharing practical information, offering advice on training and giving race tips. What you're doing now is conditioning your brain and body to last for longer periods. You'll be applying exactly the same principles to these longer distances as those that underpinned the training for your 5K race: slow, steady, gradual increases in your weekly mileage, in particular your weekly long run.

So, write your new goal in your training diary and then just go for it, confident in the belief that you can do it. The example training programme below is just one illustration of how you can do it. Please note that if you've already run a couple of 10K races and now feel it's time to start working on improving your time, then take a look at the 10K training programme in the 'experienced intermediate' section on page 92.

	monday	tuesday	wednesday
week 1	Rest day	5-min warm-up jog/walk. Stretches. 2.5-mile easy run.	Rest day
week 2	Rest day	5-min warm-up jog/walk. Stretches. 3-mile steady run.	Rest day
week 3	Rest day	5-min warm-up jog. Stretches. 3.5-mile steady run.	Rest day or swim, walk or cross-train.
week 4	Rest day	5-min warm-up jog. Stretches. 4-mile steady run.	Rest day or swim, walk or cross-train.
week 5	Rest day	5-min warm-up jog. Stretches. 4.5-mile steady run.	Rest day or swim, walk or cross-train.
week 6	Rest day	5-min warm-up jog. Stretches. 4-mile steady run, 3 x 100m at a faster pace (walk back in between).	Rest day or swim, walk or cross-train.
week 7	Rest day	5-min warm-up jog. Stretches. 4.5-mile steady run; 3 x 100m faster runs (walk back in between).	Rest day or swim, walk or cross-train.
week 8	Rest day	5-min jog and stretches. 3-mile steady run; 4–5 x 100m faster runs (walk back in between).	3-mile steady run

2.5 miles = 4 km, 3 miles = 4.8 km, 3.5 miles = 5.5 km, 4 miles = 6.5 km, 4.5 miles = 7.25 km, 5 miles = 8 km, 6 miles = 9.5 km, 7 miles = 11.25 km

notes

- The week can be rotated to suit people's schedules – I've just assumed that the first day of a standard working week is good for a rest day, and that many people will have more time for the longer run and to get to a park or an off-road route at the weekend.

- I've introduced a brisker pace in the strides just to wake up the faster twitch muscles a bit, give some variety and make the steady running feel easier.

- In the Thursday runs, I'm trying to get the heart rate up and intensify cardiovascular training by including some hills. Try and maintain your pace on the hills, even though it will feel – and be – harder; this will make you stronger, as well as add a bit of variety. If hills are hard to find, pick a short stretch to pick up the pace a bit.

thursday	friday	saturday	sunday
5-min jog. Stretches. 3-mile steady run.	Swim, walk or cross-train.	Rest day	3-mile easy/steady run.
5-min jog. Stretches. 4-mile steady run, including a couple of good hills, if possible. Maintain as much good form and speed up the hill as possible.	Swim, walk or cross-train.	Rest day	4-mile steady run off-road, if possible.
5-min jog. Stretches. 4-mile steady run, including a couple of good hills, if possible; maintain as much good form and speed up the hill as possible.	Swim, walk or cross-train.	Rest day	5-mile steady run off-road, if possible.
5-min jog. Stretches. 5-mile steady run, including a couple of good hills. Maintain as much good form and speed up the hill as possible.	2-mile easy run. Stretches.	Rest day	6-mile steady run in the park or off-road.
5-min jog. Stretches. 5-mile steady run, including a couple of good hills. Maintain as much good form and speed up the hill as possible.	2 to 3-mile easy run. Stretches	Rest day	7-mile steady run off-road
5-min jog. Stretches. 6-mile steady run, including a couple of good hills. Maintain as much good form and speed up the hill as possible.	2 to 3-mile easy run. Stretches	Rest day	7-mile steady run off-road
5-min jog. Stretches. 5-mile steady run, including a couple of good hills. Maintain as much good form and speed up the hill as possible.	2-mile easy run. Stretches	Rest day	6-mile steady run off-road
Rest day	2 to 3-mile easy run; 4 x 100m faster runs.	Rest day	**RACE DAY**

how to train for a half-marathon

Okay, it may seem like an enormous difference between a 10K and a half-marathon, given that at 21K (or 13.1 miles, if you prefer), the half-marathon is double the distance. However, rest assured that in reality there really isn't such a massive jump between the two.

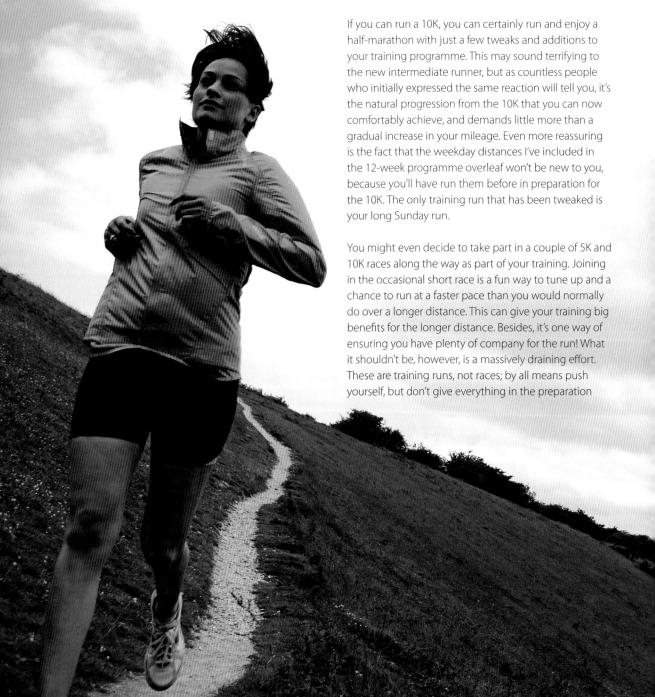

If you can run a 10K, you can certainly run and enjoy a half-marathon with just a few tweaks and additions to your training programme. This may sound terrifying to the new intermediate runner, but as countless people who initially expressed the same reaction will tell you, it's the natural progression from the 10K that you can now comfortably achieve, and demands little more than a gradual increase in your mileage. Even more reassuring is the fact that the weekday distances I've included in the 12-week programme overleaf won't be new to you, because you'll have run them before in preparation for the 10K. The only training run that has been tweaked is your long Sunday run.

You might even decide to take part in a couple of 5K and 10K races along the way as part of your training. Joining in the occasional short race is a fun way to tune up and a chance to run at a faster pace than you would normally do over a longer distance. This can give your training big benefits for the longer distance. Besides, it's one way of ensuring you have plenty of company for the run! What it shouldn't be, however, is a massively draining effort. These are training runs, not races; by all means push yourself, but don't give everything in the preparation race. Burning yourself out at this point will only jeopardise your performance at the very event for which you've put in so much effort. Come away feeling as though you've worked hard, but that you'll recover quickly and learn from the experience, having enjoyed the race without putting yourself under any pressure.

BUILD UP YOUR MUSCULAR STRENGTH

At this stage, you'll want to incorporate some weight-lifting and core strength work into your weekly routine. Strengthening your muscles to support the hard work you're putting your body through is a preventative measure – a means of reducing injury risk, but also speeding up recovery from hard training and from injury if you're unfortunate enough to sustain one. Plus, increasing your muscular strength increases your endurance capability. (See page 34, Chapter 3, Taking care of your body.)

As your distances creep up, your rest days become even more important, cutting some well-earned slack during which your body gets a chance to rest, recover and carry out essential repairs to its muscles, tendons and ligaments. If you can do some of your distance training on low-impact surfaces such as grass or dirt tracks, rather than tarmac and paving slabs, so much the better for your joints. In general, I try to do 70–75% of my running on softer surfaces. This helps recovery, but also means your lower limb muscles and feet are working harder for the same distance, so it will feel that much easier when you race on the road. Plus, it's more fun!

FIND YOUR TRAINING ZONE

Now that your training is steadily progressing, you'll be getting a good idea of your optimum speed. It's important to track your pace over the months of training so that you go into the race with a pretty clear idea of what it should be on the day. Use a sports watch to monitor it – this will act as a useful energy-conserving device and stop you from going out too fast too early. A heart rate monitor watch can help further; to use one properly, you need to know what your maximum heart rate (MHR) is so that you can determine your training zones. This is fairly easy to do. You can get tested in a laboratory, but you can also just

go out and run as hard as you can and see what your MHR is. For example, on a day when you are rested and feeling good, go out, warm up well then run something like 5 runs of 3–5 mins hard, with a 2/3-minute jog/walk in between. When you look back at the recorded heart rates you'll see the maximum that you reached, probably in the later repetitions. Once you know your MHR, you can then work out the training zones for recovery runs, steady runs and hard runs, and your training will become more efficient. There are a number of good quality heart rate monitors out there – I use the Nike Triax Elite, which is comfortable and has all the functions I need. It also allows me to download my training sessions from the watch to my computer after each run so that I can analyse it and assess how the session went.

LISTEN TO YOUR BODY

Don't stress if you pick up a virus or a niggle and need to take a couple of days off; runners can become obsessively fixated on their training programme – very occasionally, dare I say, to the exclusion of common sense. If you don't feel great, don't risk it; you'll only put yourself, quite literally, out of the running for even longer. What's a couple of days of no training compared with months off due to ignoring the warning signs? Anyway, if you've picked up an injury and you're off the road, chances are you'll be able to keep your fitness levels up by swimming or cycling while your injury heals. Plus, as I have discovered so many times over, the time away only goes to make your running feel even more special and appreciated when you get back, which, in turn, boosts your performances. Obviously, take advice from a clinical professional. If push comes to shove and you do find yourself having to miss out on the half-marathon you had set your heart on running, set your sights on the next one. It's no bad thing to have extra time – you'll be even better prepared for it. Rushing to be ready for something with insufficient time or strength is dangerous as well as physically and mentally debilitating.

Lastly, test anything new – clothing or new energy drinks – in training. You'll have enough to consider on race day without wondering how your stomach will react to a totally untested brand of drink.

And don't forget, stretching is a given before and after every run!

'new intermediates' half-marathon training programme

By now you've put a huge tick in the box alongside '10K' on your list of achievements, your confidence is growing and you may well have the next distance runner's milestone in your sights: the half-marathon. This programme shows how to gradually take your training up a gear and, for the first time, includes a training method known as 'fartlek'. This means 'speed play' in Swedish: bursts of high-intensity effort alternating with less strenuous intervals, either planned or random to suit yourself.

	monday	tuesday	wednesday
week 1	Rest day	6-mile steady run.	Active rest: Walk or swim, plus core strength exercises and stretching at home.
week 2	Rest day	6-mile steady run.	Active rest: Walk or swim, plus core strength exercises and stretching at home.
week 3	Rest day	6-mile steady run.	Active rest: Walk or swim, plus core strength exercises and stretching at home.
week 4	Rest day	6-mile steady run. 3 x 100m strides (walk back to recover).	Option: Active rest, or 2-mile jog and core strength programme.
week 5	Rest day	6-mile steady run. 4 x 150m strides (walk or jog back to recover).	Active rest: Walk or swim, plus core strength exercises and stretching at home.
week 6	Rest day	6-mile steady run. 4 x 150m strides. (walk or jog back to recover).	Option: Active rest or 3-mile jog and core strength programme.
week 7	Rest day	6-mile run, split over: 2 miles easy, 2 miles tempo (at a sustained, faster-than-target-race pace), 2 miles easy.	Active rest: Walk or swim, plus core strength exercises and stretching at home.
week 8	Rest day	7-mile run split over: 2 miles easy; 3 miles tempo; 2 miles easy.	Option: Active rest or 3-mile jog and core strength programme.
week 9	Rest day	7-mile run split over: 2 miles easy; 3 miles tempo; 2 miles easy.	Active rest: Walk or swim, plus core strength exercises and stretching at home.
week 10	Rest day	7-mile steady run.	Option: Active rest or 3-mile jog and core strength programme.
week 11	Rest day	7-mile run, split over: 2 miles easy; 3 miles tempo; 2 miles easy.	Active rest: Walk or swim, plus core strength exercises and stretching at home.
week 12	Rest day	5-mile steady run. 4 x 100m strides (walk back to recover), 1-mile jog.	Active rest: Walk or swim. Core strength exercises at home.

1 mile = 1.6 km, 2 miles = 3.25 km, 3 miles = 4.8 km, 4 miles = 6.5 km, 5 miles = 8 km, 6 miles = 9.5 km, 7 miles = 11.25 km, 8 miles = 12.9 km

I've assumed that people starting this would have already followed the previous 10K programme, or something similar. Again, I've made Monday the rest day, on the basis that many people prefer to do the long run on a Sunday, but the week can be rotated to make any day the start.

Tip: For the Saturday fartlek session, run with friends and take turns picking the length of pace pick-ups. Or ask a friend to come on a bike and blow a whistle for each change. Use the same route for the tempo (see page 104) part of your Tuesday run so that you can see if you get further.

thursday	friday	saturday	sunday
5-mile steady run.	Rest day. Core strength exercises and stretches.	2-mile jog. Stretching. On a 200–250m hill, run 2 sets of 5 hills, focusing on good form. Jog down to recover between runs. Walk between sets. 1- to 2-mile jog.	8-mile steady run, off-road if possible. Practise drinking during.
6-mile steady run.	Rest day. Core strength exercises and stretches.	1-mile jog. Stretching. 35 mins of fartlek: set off at easy pace and pick the pace up for short bursts of 20 secs–2 mins (slow down to easy pace to recover). 2-mile jog.	9-mile steady run, off-road if possible. Practise drinking during.
6-mile steady run.	Rest day. Core strength exercises and stretches.	2-mile jog. Stretching. On a 200–250m hill, run 2 sets of 6 hills, focusing on good form. Jog down to recover between runs. Walk between sets. 2-mile jog.	10-mile steady run, off-road if possible. Practise drinking during.
6-mile steady run.	Rest day. Core strength exercises and stretches.	1-mile jog. 40 mins of fartlek as per week 2. 1-mile jog.	11-mile steady run, off-road if possible. Practise drinking during.
7-mile steady run.	Rest day. Core strength exercises and stretches.	2-mile jog. Stretching. On a 200–250m hill, run 3 sets of 5 hill runs, focusing on good form. Jog down to recover between runs. Walk between sets.1–2-mile jog.	12-mile steady run, off-road if possible. Practise drinking during.
7-mile steady run.	Rest day. Core strength exercises and stretches.	1-mile jog. 40 mins of fartlek. 1-mile jog.	12-mile steady run, off-road if possible. Practise drinking during.
7-mile steady run.	Rest day. Core strength exercises and stretches.	2-mile jog. Stretching. On a 200–250m hill, run 3 sets of 5 hills focusing on good form. Jog down to recover between runs. Walk between sets. 2-mile jog.	13-mile steady run, off-road if possible. Practise drinking during.
7 to 8-mile steady run.	Rest day. Core strength exercises and stretches.	1-mile jog. 45 mins of fartlek. 1-mile jog.	14-mile steady run, off-road if possible. Practise drinking during.
8-mile steady run.	Rest day. Core strength exercises and stretches.	2-mile jog. Stretching. On a 200–250m hill, run 3 sets of 5 hills focusing on good form. Jog down to recover. Walk between sets. 2-mile jog.	14-mile steady run, off road if possible. Practise drinking during.
7 to 8-mile steady run.	Rest day. Core strength exercises and stretches.	1-mile jog. 40 mins of fartlek. 1-mile jog.	13-mile steady run, off road if possible.
6-mile steady run. 3 to 4 x 100m strides.	Rest day. Core strength exercises and stretches.	2-mile jog. Stretching. On a 200–250m hill. Run 2 sets of 6 hills focusing on good form. Jog down to recover. Walk between sets. 2-mile jog.	10-mile steady run, off-road if possible.
5-mile easy run.	Rest day. Core strength exercises and stretches.	Rest day	**RACE HALF-MARATHON**

9 miles = 14.5 km, 10 miles = 16 km, 11 miles = 17.7 km, 12 miles = 19.3 km, 13 miles = 21 km, 14 miles = 22.5 km

'new intermediates' marathon training programme

I've worked on the assumption that you've already done the training for the 10K, plus the fitness training for the half-marathon, and that you're running four days a week. My aim is to get you to run around your first marathon comfortably and finish it with a smile on your face!

	monday	tuesday	wednesday
week 1	Rest day	40-min steady run.	Rest. 30 minutes of home core strength and conditioning exercises.
week 2	Rest day	40-min steady run. 3 x 100m strides (see page 104), walk back to recover.	Rest. 30 minutes of home core strength and conditioning exercises.
week 3	Rest day	45-min steady run. 3 x 100m strides (walk back to recover).	Rest. 30 minutes of home core strength and conditioning exercises.
week 4	Rest day	45-min steady run. Faster-than-target-race pace, but you should be able to talk. 3 x 100m strides.	Rest. 30 minutes of home core strength and conditioning exercises.
week 5	Rest day	50-min steady run. 3 x 100m strides.	Rest. 30 minutes of home core strength and conditioning exercises.
week 6	Rest day	50-min steady run. 3 x 100m strides.	Rest. 30 minutes of home core strength and conditioning exercises.
week 7	Rest day	55-min steady run. 3 x 100m strides.	Rest. 30 minutes of home core strength and conditioning exercises.
week 8	Rest day	55-min steady run. 3 x 100m strides.	Rest. 30 minutes of home core strength and conditioning exercises.
week 9	Rest day	60-min steady run. 3 x 100m strides.	Rest. 30 minutes of home core strength and conditioning exercises.
week 10	Rest day	55-min steady run. 3 x 100m strides.	Rest. 30 minutes of home core strength and conditioning exercises.
week 11	Rest day	45-min steady run. 4 x 100m strides.	Rest. 30 minutes of home core strength and conditioning exercises.
week 12	Rest day	30-min easy run. 4 x 100m strides.	Rest. 30 minutes of home core strength and conditioning exercises.

8 miles = 12.9 km, 9 miles = 14.5 km, 10 miles = 16 km, 11 miles = 17.7 km, 12 miles = 19.3 km, 13 miles = 21 km, 14 miles = 22.5 km, 15 miles = 24 km

I've expressed runs as time taken, rather than distance – except for the long Sunday run, as people's target times will vary. Aim to get up to 80–85% of your target: e.g. if it's 4 hours or 4 hours 15 minutes, build up to a long run of 3 hours 30 minutes. Ask the family to come on bikes and plan to get an energy drink and/or snack at least a couple of times. You'll gain confidence in your ability to do it without draining the tank. On race day, sheer inspiration and adrenaline will get you through the last few miles. Stretching before and after is a given. By all means rejig the week's schedule to suit social commitments.

thursday	friday	saturday	sunday
40-min steady run.	Rest. 30 minutes of home core strength and conditioning exercises.	30-min off-road run: try and include some testing hills, if possible.	8 to 10-mile long run.
50-min steady run.	Rest. 30 minutes of home core strength and conditioning exercises.	40-min off-road run: try and include some testing hills, if possible.	12-mile long run.
60-min steady run.	Rest. 30 minutes of home core strength and conditioning exercises.	45-min off-road run: try and include some testing hills, if possible.	14-mile long run.
70-min steady/ easy run.	Rest. 30 minutes of home core strength and conditioning exercises.	50-min off-road run: try and include some testing hills, if possible.	15-mile long run.
75-min steady/easy run.	Rest. 30 minutes of home core strength and conditioning exercises.	55-min off-road run: try and include some testing hills if possible.	16-mile long run.
80-min steady/easy run.	Rest. 30 minutes of home core strength and conditioning exercises.	60-min off-road run: try and include some testing hills, if possible.	17-mile long run.
90-min steady/easy run.	Rest. 30 minutes of home core strength and conditioning exercises.	60-min off-road run: try and include some testing hills, if possible.	18-mile long run.
90-min steady/easy run.	Rest. 30 minutes of home core strength and conditioning exercises.	60-min off-road run: try and include some testing hills, if possible.	20 to 21-mile long run.
80-min steady/easy run.	Rest. 30 minutes of home core strength and conditioning exercises.	60-min off-road run: try and include some testing hills, if possible.	18-mile long run.
70-min steady/ easy run.	Rest. 30 minutes of home core strength and conditioning exercises.	50-min off-road run: try and include some testing hills if possible.	15-mile long run.
50-min steady/easy run.	Rest. 30 minutes of home core strength and conditioning exercises.	30-min steady run off-road.	8 to 10-mile long run. Some strides.
20-min easy jog. 4 x 100m strides.	Option: Rest or 15-min jog, if preferred. Stretching.	Rest day	**RACE DAY**

16 miles = 25.7 km, 17 miles = 27.3 km, 18 miles = 29 km, 19 miles = 30.5 km, 20 miles = 32 km, 21 miles = 34 km

'experienced intermediates' improve-your-10K training programme

Congratulations! You've moved beyond the 'new intermediate' stage and by now will have completed a 10K, and maybe a half-marathon. You may even have completed a marathon and, for your next goal, be looking to improve your time. Either way, you'll probably be regularly running around 20–40 miles a week, including a weekly long run of 8–15 miles. But if your dream is to improve your times, steadily bettering each personal best (PB) as you get stronger and faster, then you'll almost certainly be starting to think about doing a few things differently. Firstly, you'll be working on increasing your weekly mileage; secondly, you'll be weaving into it some higher intensity speed work. The main added ingredients are the tempo run, a shorter-than-race-distance run of 20–45 minutes' duration that you do at a comfortably hard pace, just on the threshold of manageability, and shorter speed work sessions such as a fartlek or hill reps. These training sessions are not only fun to do, they will quickly show their usefulness in your fitness and race times.

The specific distances required of you in training will obviously depend on the race you've got your eye on. Have a look at the following tables: they are illustrations that I've put together of training programmes for the 10K, half-marathon and the marathon for anyone who is well beyond a rookie runner and heading towards the 'advanced' category.

	monday	tuesday	wednesday
week 1	Rest day	1-mile jog warm-up. Stretches. 4-mile tempo run. 1-mile jog.	Strength day: 10-minute jog/cross-train warm-up. 40 minutes weights programme (Chap 3). Stretch. Optional short jog afterwards.
week 2	Rest day	1-mile jog warm-up. Stretches. 4-mile tempo run. 1-mile jog.	Strength day: 10-minute jog/cross-train warm-up. 40 minutes weights programme (Chap 3). Stretch. Optional short jog afterwards.
week 3	Rest day	1-mile jog warm-up. Stretches. 5-mile tempo run. 1-mile jog.	Strength day: 10-minute jog/cross-train warm-up. 40 minutes weights programme (Chap 3). Stretch. Optional short jog afterwards.
week 4	Rest day	1-mile jog warm-up. Stretches. 5-mile tempo run. 1-mile jog.	Strength day: 10-minute jog/cross-train warm-up. 40 minutes weights programme (Chap 3). Stretch. Optional short jog afterwards.
week 5	Rest day	1-mile jog warm-up. Stretches. 5-mile tempo run. 1-mile jog.	Strength day: 10-minute jog/cross-train warm-up. 40 minutes weights programme (Chap 3). Stretch. Optional short jog afterwards.
week 6	Rest day	1-mile jog warm-up. Stretches. 5.5-mile tempo run. 1-mile jog.	Strength day: 10-minute jog/cross-train warm-up. 40 minutes weights programme (Chap 3). Stretch. Optional short jog afterwards.
week 7	Rest day	1-mile jog warm-up. Stretches. 5-mile tempo run. 1-mile jog.	Strength day: 10-minute jog/cross-train warm-up. 40 minutes weights programme (Chap 3). Stretch. Optional short jog afterwards.
week 8	Rest day	1-mile jog. Stretches. 3-mile, good-pace run. 4 or 5 x 100m faster runs (walk back to recover). 1-mile jog.	3 to 4-mile steady run. 4 x 100m strides.

1 mile = 1.6 km, 2 miles = 3.25 km, 3 miles = 4.8 km, 4 miles = 6.5 km, 5 miles = 8 km, 5.5 miles = 8.8 km, 6 miles = 9.5 km, 7 miles = 11.25 km,

notes

- The week can be rotated to suit you; I've just assumed that the first day of a standard working week is good as a rest day, and that people may have more time for the longer run and to find an off-road route at the weekend.

- I've introduced more instances of faster pace in the tempo run, hill reps and 3-minute faster reps and, also, more strides after your runs to keep the faster twitch muscles ticking over and make the steady running and the race itself feel easier.

- The biggest change is the addition of weights/strength training from Chapter 3. Starting with one weekly session and then building to two, be sure to target different muscle areas in each session. Choose two different weights programmes each week, e.g. either A and B, or B and C, or A and C. (See weights section, page 55.)

- Although I mention stretching as part of your warm-up each time, don't forget that you must, without fail, stretch after each and every run in order to help guard against injury.

thursday	friday	saturday	sunday
1-mile jog. Stretch. 15 hill reps of 200–250m (jog down to recover): do 3 sets of 5, and walk down after each set. 1-mile jog.	45 mins of home strength and core conditioning.	5-mile easy run.	8 to 10-mile steady off-road run.
1-mile jog. Stretch. **Either** 35 mins fartlek. **Or** 6 x 3 mins hard run on road/good grass (2-min jog/walk recovery). 1-mile jog.	45 mins of home strength and core conditioning.	5-mile easy run.	10-mile off-road run.
1-mile jog. Stretch. Hill reps as before. 1-mile jog.	Gym: 40 mins of weights programme.	6-mile easy run. 2 to 3 pick-up strides to finish.	10-mile off-road run.
1-mile jog. Stretch. **Either** 40 mins fartlek. **Or** 8 x 3 mins hard run on road/good grass (2-min jog/walk to recover). 1-mile jog.	Gym: 40 mins of weights programme.	6-mile easy run, with a few strides afterwards.	10-mile off-road run.
1-mile jog. Stretch. Hill reps as before. Focus on good form and knee lift. 1-mile jog.	Gym: 40 mins of weights programme.	6-mile easy run. Strides to finish.	10-mile off-road run.
1-mile jog. Stretch. **Either** 40 mins fartlek. **Or** 8 x 3 mins hard run on road/good grass (2-min jog/walk to recover). 1-mile jog.	Gym: 40 mins of weights programme.	6-mile easy run. Strides to finish.	10-mile off-road run.
1-mile jog. Hill reps as before. 1-mile jog.	Gym: 40 mins of weights programme.	5-mile easy run. 4 x 150m strides to finish.	8-mile off-road run.
Core strength and conditioning at home.	2 to 3-mile easy run. 4 x 100m faster runs.	Rest day	**RACE DAY**

8 miles = 12.9 km, 9 miles = 14.5 km, 10 miles = 16 km

'experienced intermediates' improve-your-half-marathon programme

I've worked on the assumption that if you're about to embark on this half-marathon training schedule, you'll already have followed the previous half marathon programme, or trained according to something similar.

	monday	tuesday	wednesday
week 1	Active rest day Gym: 40 to 45 mins of Weights Session A. Don't forget the abs!	1-mile jog. 6-mile tempo run. 1-mile jog.	6-mile easy run.
week 2	Gym: 40 to 45 mins of Weights Session A.	1-mile jog. 6-mile tempo run. 1-mile jog.	6-mile easy run.
week 3	Gym: 40 to 45 mins of Weights Session A.	1-mile jog. 6-mile tempo run. 1-mile jog.	6-mile easy run.
week 4	Gym: 40 to 45 mins of Weights Session A.	1-mile jog. 7-mile tempo run. 1-mile jog.	6-mile easy run. Core strength and conditioning programme.
week 5	Gym: 40 to 45 mins of Weights Session A.	2-mile jog. 7-mile tempo run. 1-mile jog.	6-mile easy run. Core strength and conditioning programme.
week 6	Gym: 40 to 45 mins of Weights Session A.	2-mile jog. 6-mile tempo run. 1-mile jog.	6-mile easy run. Core strength and conditioning programme.
week 7	Gym: 40 to 45 mins of Weights Session A.	2-mile jog. Fartlek: 2 miles faster than race pace, 2 miles slower but still running, 2 miles faster, 2 miles slower.	6-mile easy run. Core strength and conditioning programme.
week 8	Gym: 40 to 45 mins of Weights Session A.	1-mile jog. 7-mile tempo run. 1-mile jog.	7-mile easy run. Core strength and conditioning programme.
week 9	Gym: 40 to 45 mins of Weights Session A.	2-mile jog. Mixed tempo run: 2 miles faster than goal pace, 1 mile slower, 3 miles faster. 1-mile jog.	6-mile easy run. Core strength and conditioning programme.
week 10	Gym: 40 to 45 mins of Weights Session A.	1-mile jog. 7-mile tempo run.	7-mile easy run. Core strength and conditioning programme.
week 11	Gym: 40 to 45 mins of Weights Session A.	1-mile jog. 5-mile tempo run. 1-mile jog.	6-mile easy run. Core strength and conditioning programme.
week 12	Core strength and conditioning at home.	5-mile steady run. 4 x 100m strides (walk back to recover). 1-mile jog.	Active rest: Walk or swim. Core exercises at home.

1 mile = 1.6 km, 2 miles = 3.25 km, 3 miles = 4.8 km, 4 miles = 6.5 km, 5 miles = 8 km, 6 miles = 9.5 km, 7 miles = 11.25 km, 8 miles = 12.9 km,

I've allowed for two rest days on a Monday and Friday, but still included some gym work. Again, the week can be rotated any way that works around work/family commitments.
Tip: For the Saturday fartlek session, run with friends and take turns choosing the length of pace pick-ups. Or get your partner/friend/kids to come with you on a bike and blow a whistle or ring a bell for each change of pace.
Tip: Use the same route for the tempo section of your Tuesday run so that you can see if you get any further the next time. Stretching is, of course, a given before and after every run.

thursday	friday	saturday	sunday
1 to 2-mile jog. 5 x 4-min hard runs (with HR above 80%). 2 to 3-min slow-jog recovery between each. 1 to 2-mile jog.	Rest day. Core strength exercises and stretches.	2-mile jog. Stretching. On a 200–250m hill, run 3 sets of 5 hills with good form. Jog down to recover and walk between sets.	10-mile steady off-road run. Practise drinking during.
1 to 2-mile jog. 6 x 4-min hard runs. 2-minute slow-jog recovery between each. 1 to 2-mile jog.	Rest day. Weights Session B or C.	1-mile jog. Stretching. 40 mins of fartlek: set off at easy pace and pick the pace up for 20 secs–2 mins. Slow down to easy pace until you recover, and then go again. 2-mile jog.	10-mile steady off-road run. Practise drinking during.
1 to 2-mile jog. 5 x 5-min hard runs. 2 to 3-min slow-jog recovery between each. 1 to 2-mile jog.	Rest day. Weights Session B or C.	2-mile jog. Stretching. On a 200–250m hill, run 2 sets of 8 hills with good form. Jog down to recover and walk between sets. 2-mile jog.	11-mile steady off-road run. Practise drinking during.
1 to 2-mile jog. 5 x 5-min hard runs. 2 to 3-min slow-jog recovery between each. 1 to 2-mile jog.	Rest day. Weights Session B or C.	1-mile jog. 45 minutes fartlek, as per week 2. 1-mile jog.	12-mile steady off-road run. Practise drinking during.
1 to 2-mile jog. Hard runs (in mins): 2, 3, 4, 5, 5, 4, 3, 2, with 2-min slow jog recovery in between each. 1 to 2-mile jog.	Rest day. Weights Session B or C.	2-mile jog. Stretching. On a 200–250m hill, run 2 sets of 8 hills focusing on good form. Jog down to recover and walk between sets. 1 to 2-mile jog.	12-mile steady off-road run. Practise drinking during.
1 to 2-mile jog. 5 x 5-min hard runs. 2-min jog recovery between each. 1 to 2-mile jog.	Rest day. Weights Session B or C.	1-mile jog. 45 mins of fartlek. 1-mile jog.	13-mile steady off-road run. Practise drinking during.
1 to 2-mile jog. 5 x 6-min hard runs. 2 min 30 sec jog recovery between each. 1 to 2-mile jog.	Rest day. Weights Session B or C.	2-mile jog. Stretching. On a 200–250m hill, run 15 hills focusing on good form. Jog down to recover. 2-mile jog.	14-mile steady run, off-road if possible. Practise drinking during.
1 to 2-mile jog. 5 x 6-min hard runs. 2 min 30 secs jog recovery between each. 1 to 2-mile jog.	Rest day. Weights Session B or C.	1-mile jog. 45 mins of fartlek. 1-mile jog	15-mile off-road run. Drink during.
1 to 2-mile jog. 5 x 3-min sustained runs at 70–80% max HR (feels fast, but comfortable). 1 to 2-mile jog.	Rest day. Weights Session B or C.	Rest day.	10K race. Warm up well before and jog a mile slowly afterwards.
7 to 8-mile steady run.	Rest day. Weights Session B or C.	1-mile jog. 45 mins of fartlek. 1-mile jog.	14-mile steady run, off-road if possible.
6-mile steady run. 3 or 4 x 100m strides.	Rest day. Weights Session B or C.	2-mile jog. Stretching. On a 200–250m hill, run 2 sets of 6 hills focusing on good form. Jog down to recover and walk between sets. 2-mile jog.	11-mile steady/ easy run, off-road if possible.
5-mile easy run.	3-mile easy run. Core strength and conditioning at home.	Rest day.	**RACE HALF-MARATHON**

9 miles = 14.5 km, 10 miles = 16 km, 11 miles = 17.7 km, 12 miles = 19.3 km, 13 miles = 21 km, 14 miles = 22.5 km, 15 miles = 24 km

'experienced intermediates' improve-your-marathon programme

	monday	tuesday	wednesday
week 1	Rest day. Gym weights programme: Session A for the week.	2-mile jog. 6-mile tempo run. 1-mile jog.	7-mile steady/easy run.
week 2	Rest day. Gym weights programme: Session A for the week.	2-mile jog. 6-mile tempo run. 1-mile jog.	8-mile steady/easy run.
week 3	Rest day. Gym weights programme: Session A for the week.	2-mile jog. 7-mile tempo run. 1-mile jog.	9-mile steady/easy run.
week 4	Rest day. Gym weights programme: Session A for the week.	2-mile jog. 7-mile tempo run. 1-mile jog.	10-mile steady/easy run.
week 5	Rest day. Gym weights programme: Session A for the week.	2-mile jog. 7-mile tempo run. 1-mile jog.	10-mile steady/easy run.
week 6	Rest day. Gym weights programme: Session A for the week.	2-mile jog. 6-mile tempo run. 1-mile jog.	10-mile steady/easy run.
week 7	Rest day. Gym weights programme: Session A for the week.	2-mile jog. 6-mile tempo run. 1-mile jog.	10-mile steady/easy run.
week 8	Rest day. Gym weights programme: Session A for the week.	2-mile jog. 7-mile tempo run. 1-mile jog.	11-mile steady/easy run.
week 9	Rest day. Gym weights programme: Session A for the week.	2-mile jog. 7-mile tempo run. 1-mile jog.	11-mile steady/easy run.
week 10	Rest day. Gym weights programme: Session A for the week.	2-mile jog. 7-mile tempo run. 1-mile jog.	10 to 12 mile steady/easy run.
week 11	Rest day. Gym weights programme: Session A for the week.	2-mile jog. 7-mile tempo run. 1-mile jog.	10-mile steady/easy run.
week 12	Rest day. Gym weights programme: Session A for the week.	2-mile jog. 7-mile tempo run. 1-mile jog.	10-mile steady/easy run.
week 13	Rest day. Gym weights programme: Session A for the week.	2-mile jog. 7-mile tempo run. 1-mile jog.	10 to 12-mile steady/easy run.
week 14	Rest day. Gym weights programme: Session A for the week.	2-mile jog. 6-mile tempo run. 1-mile jog.	9-mile steady/easy run.
week 15	Rest day. Home core strength and conditioning	2-mile jog. 5-mile tempo run. 1-mile jog.	7-mile steady/easy run.
week 16	Rest day. Core strength and conditioning.	6-mile easy run. 4 x 100m strides.	5-mile easy run. 4 x 100m strides

1 mile = 1.6 km, 2 miles = 3.25 km, 3 miles = 4.8 km, 4 miles = 6.5 km, 5 miles = 8 km, 6 miles = 9.5 km, 7 miles = 11.25 km, 8 miles = 12.9 km, 9 miles = 14.5 km, 10 miles = 16 km, 11 miles = 17.7 km, 12 miles = 19.3 km, 13 miles = 21 km, 14 miles = 22.5 km, 15 miles = 24 km, 16 miles = 25.7 km, 17 miles = 27.3 km 18 miles = 29 km, 19 miles = 30.5 km, 20 miles = 32 km, 21 miles = 34 km, 22 miles = 35.5 km

thursday	friday	saturday	sunday
7-mile steady run.	Gym weights programme: Session B for the week.	8-mile good-paced run, including some hills.	12-mile long run off-road if possible.
7-mile steady run.	Gym weights programme: Session B for the week.	9-mile good-paced run – try and include some hilly terrain.	14-mile long run off-road if possible.
2-mile warm-up, 1-mile cool-down. 5 x 5 mins of hard effort (80–85% of max HR). 2-min jog recovery between reps.	Gym weights programme: Session B for the week.	2-mile jog warm-up. 40 mins of fartlek, pick-ups from 20 secs–3 mins long. 1-mile jog.	14-mile long run off-road if possible.
2-mile warm-up, 2-mile cool-down. 5 x 5 mins of hard effort (80–85% of max HR). 2-min jog recovery between reps.	Gym weights programme: Session B for the week.	2-mile jog warm-up. 45 mins of fartlek. 1-mile jog.	16-mile long run off-road if possible.
2-mile warm-up, 2-mile cool-down. 6 x 5 mins of hard effort (80–85% of max HR). 2-min jog recovery between reps.	Gym weights programme: Session B for the week.	2-mile warm-up and cool-down. 2 sets of 8 x 250m hills. Jog down to recover. Walk between sets.	16-mile long run off-road if possible.
2-mile warm-up, 1-mile cool-down. 5 x 5 mins of hard effort (80–85% of max HR). 2-min jog recovery between reps.	Gym weights programme: Session B for the week.	Rest, if racing tomorrow. **Or** 2-mile jog warm-up. 45 mins of fartlek over hills. 1-mile jog.	10K race. **Or** 16-mile long run off-road if possible.
2-mile warm-up, 2-mile cool-down. 5 x 5 mins of hard effort (80–85% of max HR). 2-min jog recovery between reps.	Gym weights programme: Session B for the week.	Rest, if racing tomorrow. **Or** 2-mile jog warm-up. 45 mins of fartlek over hills. 1-mile jog.	10K race, if not last weekend. **Or** 18-mile long run off-road if possible.
2-mile warm-up, 2-mile cool-down. 5 x 6 mins of hard effort (80–85% of max HR). 2-min jog recovery between reps.	Gym weights programme: Session B for the week.	2-mile warm-up and cool-down. 2 sets of 8 x 250m hills. Jog down to recover. Walk between sets.	20-mile long run off-road if possible.
2-mile warm-up, 2-mile cool-down. 5 x 6 mins of hard effort (80–85% of max HR). 2-min jog recovery between reps.	Gym weights programme: Session B for the week.	2-mile warm-up. 50 mins of fartlek. 1-mile cool-down.	22-mile long run off-road if possible.
2-mile warm-up, 2-mile cool-down. 6 x 6 mins of hard effort (80–85% of max HR). 2-min jog recovery between reps.	Gym weights programme: Session B for the week.	2-mile warm-up and cool-down. 2 sets of 8 x 250m hills. Jog down to recover. Walk between sets.	18-mile long run off-road if possible.
2-mile warm-up and 2-mile cool-down. 5 x 6 mins of hard effort (80-85% of max HR), but 4 x if racing. 2-min jog between reps.	Gym weights programme: Session B for the week.	Rest, if racing. **Or** 2-mile warm-up. 45 mins of fartlek. 1-mile jog.	Half-marathon race, **Or** 18-mile long run off-road if possible.
2-mile warm-up and 2-mile cool-down. 5 x 6 mins of hard effort (80-85% of max HR), but 4 x if racing. 2-min jog between reps. 2-min jog to recover between reps.	Gym weights programme: Session B for the week.	Rest, if racing. **Or** 2-mile warm-up. 50 mins of fartlek. 1-mile jog.	Half-marathon race, **Or** 20-mile long run off-road if possible.
2-mile warm-up and 2-mile cool-down. 5 x 6 mins of hard effort (80–85% of max HR). 2-min jog between reps. 2-min jog to recover between reps.	Gym weights programme: Session B for the week.	2-mile warm-up and cool-down. 2 sets of 8 x 250m hills. Jog down to recover. Walk between sets.	18-mile long run off-road if possible.
2-mile warm-up and 2-mile cool-down. 5 x 6 mins of hard effort (80–85% of max HR). 2-min jog between reps. 2-min jog to recover between reps.	Gym weights programme: Session 2 for the week.	2-mile warm-up jog. 45 mins of fartlek. 1-mile jog.	15-mile long run off-road if possible.
2-mile warm-up and 2-mile cool-down. 5 x 4 mins of hard effort (80–85% of max HR). 2-min jog between reps. 2-min jog to recover between reps.	Home core strength and conditioning.	2-mile warm-up jog. 35 mins of fartlek. 1-mile jog.	10-mile long run off-road if possible.
3 to 4-mile jog. 4 x 100m strides.	Rest day. Core strength and conditioning.	Rest day.	**MARATHON RACE DAY**

race day tips

You've put in the hard work, you're tuned up and you're ready to race. Now all you've got to do is get it right on the day. Here are 10 tips that will contribute towards a smooth and enjoyable race.

1 You'll obviously have tried out various types of night-before suppers and pre-run breakfasts during your months of training to see what suits you best, so in the days leading up to the race just make sure you get a balanced, nutritious diet (see Chapter 9, Eat to win). Don't choose now to try experimenting – stick to what you're used to and know is safe. A week before the race, tip your protein/carbohydrate ratio in favour of carbs in order to build up fuel in your tank for the race, and make sure you take on board enough fibre to keep you regular. Speaking of fibre, don't forget that fruit and veg count as carbs just as much as pasta, rice and potatoes. No need to wildly increase your calorie intake for shorter races – over-eating will just make you feel bloated, so just switch the emphasis from protein to carbs. But in preparation for long races, ramp up your carbohydrate intake three days beforehand: the food you take on board is converted to glycogen, which is stored in the muscles and liver and will be used to power your effort in the race. You can do this either with carbohydrate drinks or bars, or choosing a larger plate of pasta or rice than normal, whichever works for you. Don't neglect your fluid balance in the build-up: you also need water in order to store carbohydrate in your muscles, so stay well hydrated. If you deplete your glycogen reserves before the finish, you'll hit the dreaded 'wall' in the race (see No. 10).

2 Have a look at a rough layout of the course so that you know where the steep hills lurk – you'll be able to take these into account in your time predictions.

3 Breakfast early enough to leave time for a loo visit before you head for the race – having to go at the venue usually means joining a lengthy Portaloo queue. Everyone will have their favourite breakfast – for some it's peanut butter on brown toast; for others it's a balanced soya smoothie. For me, since I discovered that I'm lactose intolerant, it's porridge with water, or cereal with rice milk, plus a banana and lots of honey. I also have an energy bar, some dark chocolate and green tea or my usual type of coffee (if I can't get the type I'm used to, I stick to green tea). I then sip an energy drink while I get ready to leave

for the race. I aim to drink another 500ml of my energy drink in the 60–90 minutes before the race. My alarm is always set so that I can finish eating three hours before I start my warm-up. I also make sure to prepare a recovery protein-and-energy drink for after the race, and plenty of energy bars/snacks in case it's a while before I find food.

4 Make a list well in advance before the nerves set in. Check you have everything: race number, watch, bottle of water/energy drink, mobile phone, post-race snack, towel, tissues, warm dry clothes to put on afterwards.

5 Leave plenty of time to get to the start. Arriving late means arriving flustered – the wrong state of mind before a challenge. My very first race at age 12, the National Cross-Country Championships, will forever be emblazoned on my memory. My parents got me there only half an hour before the start of the race. I then had to queue for 15 minutes for the toilets. I was stressed and didn't race as well as I wanted to. From that day on, I told my parents that my race was due to start an hour before it actually did. It can take up to half an hour to find parking and get to the start, and even though you'll have received your race number in the post, you may still have to collect your timing chip from the organisers' tent, plus you need to warm up and stretch, as well as queue for the loo. Take plastic covers or old clothes that you can throw away to keep warm at the start. For big races, your bag and clothes get loaded on to the baggage buses a while before the start, and you want to stay warm (and dry) while you wait.

6 Don't start too fast when the gun goes off. This is a mistake often made by less experienced runners: you feel great, the weather's perfect, so you hit it like a greyhound out of a trap – often together with others around you. Trouble is, you don't know their race plan: they might be more experienced than you are and are intending to run a faster pace; or they may have misjudged it, too, in which case you'll be seeing them later when you're all walking! Luckily, in big races you may find that the sheer number of runners will slow you down. If you think you're going too slowly, don't worry: stay calm and make up the time with the energy you've saved when the crowds thin out.

7 Set your watch as you cross the line and use it to make sure that you stick to your race plan: you know what your optimum pace is from training, so keep an eye on your mile splits to make sure that you have enough left in the tank to have a good finish.

8 Keep an eye out for water and energy drink stations – the big races often have signs indicating water tables ahead. You'll usually have a choice of several tables at each station, so you don't have to grab water at the first one amid the crush and chaos. Some have bottles and others cups, so practice drinking from both beforehand. Hang on to the bottle for a minute or two and take small swallows rather than big gulps, allowing the first to go down before you take the next. Most marathons also offer energy drinks at the stations; if you know this beforehand, try it so as to be sure your stomach will like it.

9 For shorter runs, water is all you require. But if you're running for more than 80–90 minutes, you'll need an additional energy drink to maintain your carbohydrate fuel system and also the balance of electrolytes (calcium, magnesium, sodium, chloride, potassium, phosphate, sulphate and bicarbonate) that your organs need in order to function. When you sweat a lot and drink a lot of water, your sodium concentration can become so diluted in your bloodstream that you start to cramp and feel dizzy, nauseous and disoriented. Confusingly, the symptoms are very similar to those associated with dehydration, so distinguishing between the two is an important job for the paramedics who attend the big races. By alternating water with an energy drink at every other table, usually from 5km (3 miles) into a marathon, you'll avoid this. And if the weather's hot, slow down while you drink – walking just for the few seconds that you're drinking will enable you to do it more efficiently with negligible loss of time.

10 'Hitting the wall' is the feeling that you've given it everything you've got and, in the process, depleted your muscle glycogen stores. What little fuel is left in the tank is running out rapidly. Generally, this is because you started out too fast; your energy stores have depleted very quickly due to inadequate nutritional preparation and carbohydrate-loading beforehand and dehydration.

Pay attention to these 10 points and you'll have a terrific race. **Enjoy the experience!**

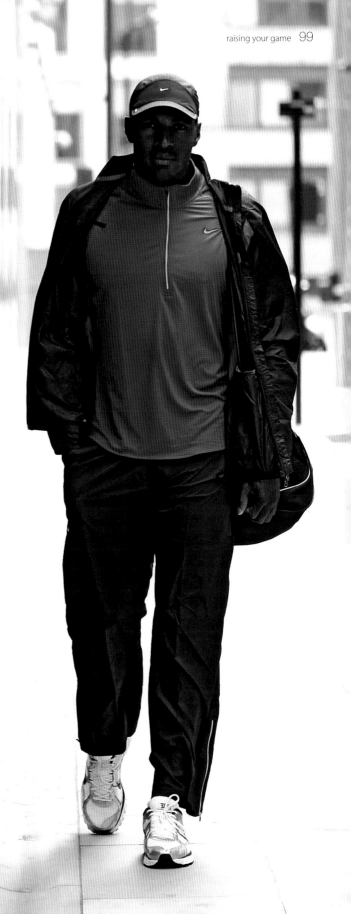

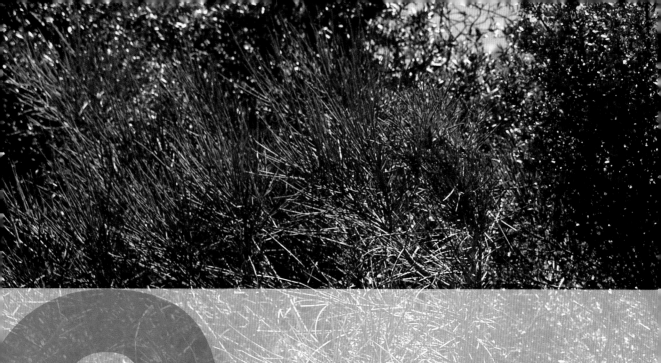

getting serious

Aiming for the top requires a different approach: smart, strategic thinking, an analytical view of your own performance, and a game plan that will give you an edge.

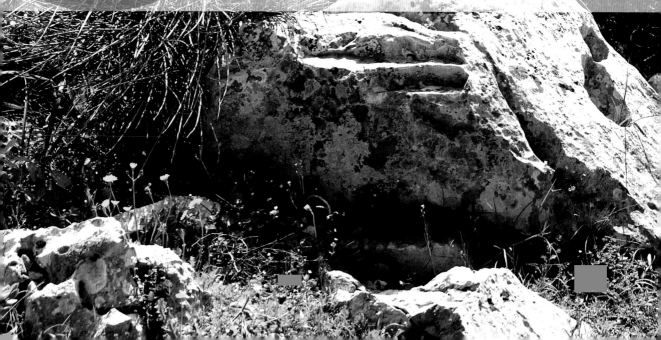

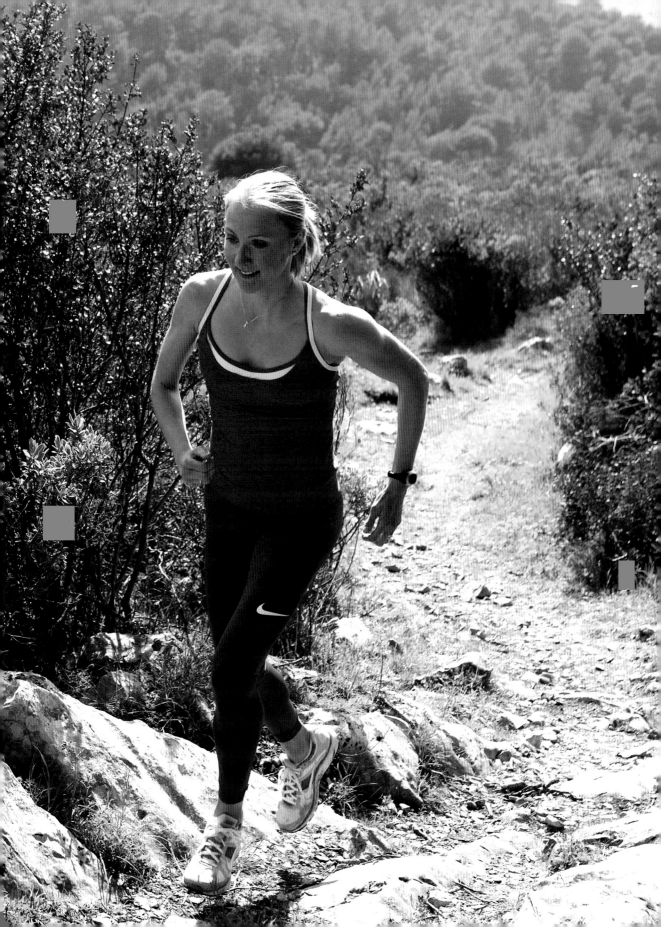

joining the élite

In Chapters 4 and 5 I looked at people who are new to running and those who have some experience. But what if you're an advanced runner who wants to get serious about your running? Who wants to run faster, get stronger and become more strategic in your training and racing?

If this describes you, then you're probably already doing one long run a week of 60–90 minutes; indeed, you may have already run a marathon and now want to improve your time. You've probably also run several races with promising results, and now have your sights set on doing a 10K in 33–50 mins; a half-marathon in 70–100 mins; or a marathon in 2hrs 40 mins–3hrs 45 mins. Training at this level is about thinking smart and being precise and selective; it starts with setting up the right circumstances for training and then getting your workload right. This is what I've found out over the years…

WATCH YOUR WEIGHT

I almost hesitate to say this, as it relies on having an accurate perception of your own body weight: if you know that you genuinely are carrying a few extra pounds, then review what you're eating. Remember, we're not talking about 'dieting' in the fashionable sense of the word – we're talking simply about cleaning up your act and making small improvements that have a cumulative effect. Giving up your takeaway muffin-and-latte habit, for example, will not only reduce your saturated fat and sugar levels, it will put money back in your wallet and take off at least 1–2kg, giving you an easier run. On the flip side, if you know that your calorie and nutritional intake is a bit low, you must be prepared to increase this in order to cope with harder, more structured training. Your body needs fuel to perform and recover well and you need to be prepared to give it adequate supplies. The food that you eat powers your running, so getting enough of the right kind is paramount. Chapter 9, Eat to win, has more detailed information on this subject.

KEEP YOUR FLUID LEVELS UP

If you're not keeping a close eye on your hydration levels while you're increasing your speed, duration and intensity, you may as well not put in all the hard work in the first place. You also need to keep a watchful eye on your electrolyte balance.

When you exercise, your body produces heat, which travels to the surface of the skin as sweat and evaporates, cooling you down and stopping you from overheating. If you don't replace the fluid you've lost, your blood volume drops and thickens. The result is that your heart rate rises as it struggles to keep blood flowing to your muscles and vital organs. One such vital organ is the biggest of all – your skin, and when this happens you simply stop sweating, effectively closing off your body heat's escape route. So, your temperature rises, bringing with it the distinct possibility of heatstroke and even unconsciousness. I've seen one scientific estimate that sweating off 2% in body weight (a state of mild dehydration) can reduce an athlete's performance by a whopping 10–20%. Big mistake if you're going for a good time, so keep sipping.

For a rough estimate of how much water a non-athlete needs, multiply your weight in kilos by .033 – the figure you get is your optimum daily intake of fluid. For someone weighing 60kg, for example, the arithmetic would look like this: 60kg x .033 = 1.98L; in other words, nearly two litres of non-caffeinated fluid per day. Runners perspire a lot more, so they need to drink a lot more – on a hot day, yet more again. As a rule of thumb, you should drink an extra litre for every hour that you run (read more on hydration in Chapter 9, Eat to win).

OPTIMISE YOUR STRIKE PATTERN

If your stride is very long and you over-stride, what you're actually doing is throwing your lead foot out so far in front of you that you land heavily on your heel. This acts as a braking mechanism, momentarily stopping you in your tracks at each stride. The resulting shock waves rippling up through your body hammer your joints and slow you down. Work on trying to ensure that your foot lands with knee slightly bent under your centre of gravity (think of your centre of gravity as an imaginary vertical line passing through your body, perpendicular to the surface on which you're running). This way, the impact can be absorbed

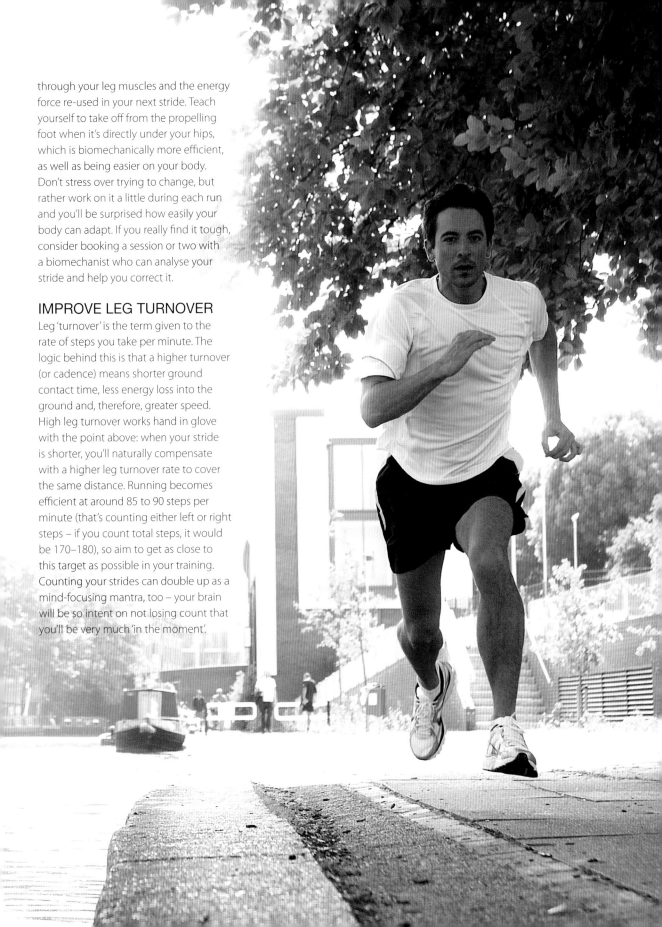

through your leg muscles and the energy force re-used in your next stride. Teach yourself to take off from the propelling foot when it's directly under your hips, which is biomechanically more efficient, as well as being easier on your body. Don't stress over trying to change, but rather work on it a little during each run and you'll be surprised how easily your body can adapt. If you really find it tough, consider booking a session or two with a biomechanist who can analyse your stride and help you correct it.

IMPROVE LEG TURNOVER

Leg 'turnover' is the term given to the rate of steps you take per minute. The logic behind this is that a higher turnover (or cadence) means shorter ground contact time, less energy loss into the ground and, therefore, greater speed. High leg turnover works hand in glove with the point above: when your stride is shorter, you'll naturally compensate with a higher leg turnover rate to cover the same distance. Running becomes efficient at around 85 to 90 steps per minute (that's counting either left or right steps – if you count total steps, it would be 170–180), so aim to get as close to this target as possible in your training. Counting your strides can double up as a mind-focusing mantra, too – your brain will be so intent on not losing count that you'll be very much 'in the moment'.

include speed work

As an experienced runner, you're probably already working on your speed and maybe even using a variety of drills; but just in case, I'll reprise the training techniques you'll need to build into your weekly routine to sharpen up.

Obviously, they vary in intensity and duration according to the distance you plan to race (see the detailed training programmes at the end of this chapter), but the principles are the same throughout.

Strides: These are short intervals of 60–200 metres, designed to improve your technique and achieve faster leg turnover. Good running technique requires a smoothly flowing forward movement with the correct knee lift and foot-strike. Get these right and they will help prevent injury, build up stamina and improve your efficiency, all of which contribute towards faster speed. Do these on a track, a path or even a field of 'good' grass, and allow the equivalent distance of jogging or walking in between to recover.

Intervals: These can be short or long, but the length and duration of the repetitions you run as part of your interval training will depend on the distance you plan to race. When preparing for a shorter race, you may do shorter, faster repetitions with, perhaps, a longer jog recovery in between, and more of them. By contrast, for marathon training you may do one session consisting of lots of shorter reps, plus one session of longer reps to boost your marathon-pace stamina. Generally, the longer the duration of the interval, the fewer the total number of repetitions per session. Fartlek training can also fall into this category, although it tends to be more of a varied-pace, threshold workout. You'll also run repetitions, but the recovery time is usually run at a slightly faster pace (more slowly than your repetition, of course, but not that much more slowly than your marathon pace).

Tempo runs: The purpose of tempo training is to build speed and stamina and it works for any distance, from 5K to the marathon. The idea is to get your body used to operating at race-pace heart rate and effort, or even a little higher, for sustained periods of time. They can be of various lengths as appropriate to the race distance for which you're training, characterised by anything from a single, hard-paced run to a few sustained-pace runs within a longer run, and are usually done once or twice a week. A classic example of a distance runner's tempo run might

be: warm-up pace for 10–15 minutes; gradual increase to a comfortably hard pace for 20–40 minutes; slower pace for the last 10–15 minutes. Someone once defined a 'challenging' phase as when you find yourself able to answer a question but unable to hold a conversation! As regards your target heart rate, aim for it to be around 80% of your max. It's easier to maintain pace and effort on a flat route; however, if you know your target race will be hilly, it makes sense to train over similar terrain.

Hill training: I have to say, I'm a big fan of hill training. Hills are a very effective means of building strength in your leg muscles and your glutes; they also give you a good opportunity to work on your form, as well as get you used to the hills you'll encounter in races. Although running hill repeats feels horribly like hard work due to the anaerobic, rather than aerobic, nature of the effort, the payoff is reduced potential for injury and faster race times thanks to increased leg strength. Find a couple of suitable hills – you need variety here, otherwise you tend to get accustomed to the same gradient; they should be runnable at a good pace rather than feel like the Matterhorn. Aim for a hard run-up time of 45–60 seconds; you can also mix in longer hills later or build them into your other runs. Concentrate on good technique, strong arm-pump and knee-lift action. The trip back down to the bottom each time is your recovery interval, so take it at a light jog – even a walk, to begin with, if you need to. Initially, your calves and Achilles will let you know that you've worked them over, so make sure you do plenty of stretching afterwards.

LONG RUNS

A 'long' run for someone whose goal is a fast 10K or half-marathon will obviously be a shorter distance than the long run done by someone preparing for a marathon. However, the principle is the same in each case: you're conditioning the muscles, joints and tendons in your feet and legs to carry you for longer; your body to push back the boundaries of fatigue and to become more efficient; and your mind to cope with the effort required to do the distance. It's estimated that your glycogen store (the fuel made from the carbs you've eaten) will power two–three hours of moderate exercise, but when you run out of glycogen you hit the wall. It's the long runs that gradually teach your body to manage its glycogen stores and usage better and enable you to extend the distance you're able to run comfortably.

The confidence you get from knowing that your body is capable of endurance running is a huge psychological advantage. Just make sure that you run them at the right pace for your training: some long runs are not meant to be done at speed, but rather to be used as a recovery run, so try to do these approx 45–75 seconds per mile slower than your estimated target race pace. Having said that, in marathon training it's sometimes good to run some long runs as a hard workout closer to your race effort – use your heart rate as a guide: the aim is gradually to teach your body to maintain that race effort for longer periods.

Have a look at the programmes that I've included in this book for how long your longer runs should be to meet your goal.

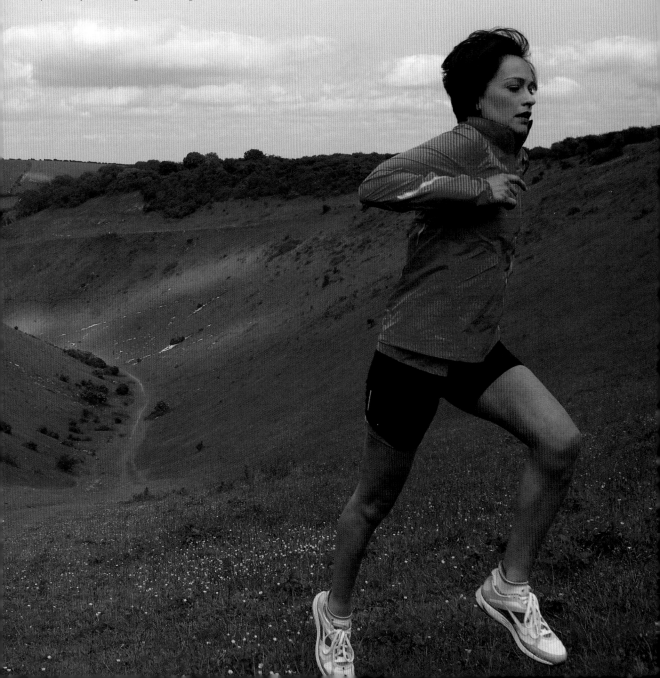

strength and conditioning

With the increased mileage, you need to build up the muscles, ligaments and tendons responsible for stabilising the joints that are put under the most stress. Our knees act as shock absorbers, lessening the impact of the running action, and they need to be bolstered with strong quadriceps and hamstrings.

Our hips also absorb shock and need to be supported by strong abductors and adductors, hip flexors and extensors, and gluteal muscles. Our ankles and feet are crucial to running and need to be supported by good upper and lower calf muscles and peroneals, as well as strong foot muscles, in order to run strongly with a smooth and efficient gait. Strong core abdominal and back muscles are vital to ensuring that all the forces produced while running are transmitted correctly and efficiently around your body. All of these need to be strengthened above and beyond the workout they

get from running. In Chapter 3, Taking care of your body, I recommended some strengthening exercises, so turn back for another look at what to incorporate in your schedule.

Lest we forget, training harder and running faster means that stretching after every run is absolutely essential; but in addition to this, a couple of times a week, after a good soak in the bath, spend half an hour stretching out all the major muscle groups. They'll reward you by performing when you most need them to respond.

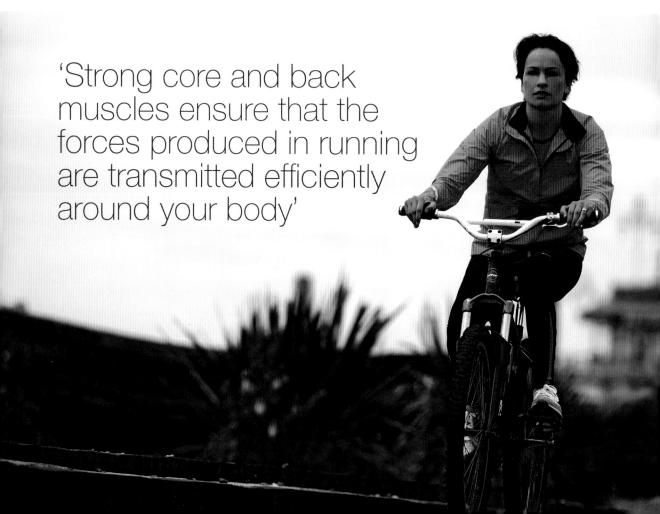

'Strong core and back muscles ensure that the forces produced in running are transmitted efficiently around your body'

RECOVERY DAYS ARE NOT OPTIONAL

Turn the concept of rest and recovery around in your head: rest is a crucial element in your training routine. It's *not* skiving off! As an advanced runner doing increased mileage, as well as a variety of interval sessions, hill training and speed work, you're courting disaster if you do hard runs day after day, piling on more and more effort without giving your body time to recover. If one day you wake up exhausted and reluctant to train after a poor night's sleep, or you feel as though your body is fighting off a low-grade virus, or your neck glands are slightly swollen and you've got a bit of a sore throat, take a look at your running diary and see whether you might have been overtraining. Then do the only sensible thing: give yourself a couple of days off and you should soon regain your fighting form. But by far the better course of action is to build a regular day of complete rest into your schedule right from the start – this will help you avoid ever getting to this point. As a rule of thumb, follow days of hard training sessions or long runs with the same number of easy days. These needn't be totally free of every kind of exercise – they can be active recovery days where you just do an easy run or a gentle swim, cycle or walk. But let me repeat: you must make sure that every 7–10 days you give yourself one complete rest day.

TAPER TRAINING

The word 'to taper' means 'to diminish', 'thin out', 'decrease to a point'. This is exactly what you do when you taper off before a race, gradually winding down your training so that you allow your body to rest, recover and build up a reserve of strength for race day. The trick is to taper off without losing your physical or mental sharpness, so the burning questions for most athletes are: 'How many days before a race should I start tapering?'; 'What should tapering look like?'; 'Should I do no exercise at all?'; 'What about just a couple of light runs?' The answer varies depending on the volume of training you've been doing up to that point, the race distance itself, and also a certain amount of experimentation to figure out what works best for you.

Before a shorter race such as a 5K or 10K, even a half-marathon, the volume of training leading into the race is not huge, so the taper period need only be 7–10 days. During this time, total volume of training will be reduced to give your legs freshness; weight training will be dropped or kept very light to improve muscle resilience; and the length and number of speed reps will decrease. This helps keep your turnover going and your mind focused, while giving your body time to recover. Personally, I prefer a couple of complete rest days before an important race, but others find their minds and bodies prefer a short, easy jog and some strides the day before. At this stage it really makes little difference how you do it – it's more important to do what you feel will get you to race day feeling good and ready to go. What I do find can work very well for shorter races is a build-up period of two to three weeks with one to two slightly less important races worked into the taper. This helps to sharpen your race instincts, as well as reduce the training volume over this period, while adding faster race intensity, more rest days and, hopefully, bags of added confidence from the good results that you've achieved in races.

Before a marathon, the taper period is longer. You should build the volume and intensity of your training to a peak about five or six weeks before the race, maintain it at that level for a couple of weeks, and then begin to taper and ease back three weeks before the race. The taper looks roughly like this: 75–80% of normal training volume three weeks before your race; 60% two weeks before it; and 30–40% in the week leading up to it. Again, mileage is reduced and weight training backs off to nothing, or very light in the week before the race. Tempo and rep session lengths are reduced slightly, but may well be run a little faster (helping with boosting your confidence, as well as leg turnover). In the week before, it's all about easy runs and some strides, with several rest days. Now is the time to concentrate on carbohydrate loading and getting down to giving lots of thought to the final details of your race strategy.

There are, of course, more ways than one to taper. It's a highly individual aspect of race preparation, and a big determining factor is what suits you personally. By its very nature, it takes a fair amount of trial and error to pin this down and is, therefore, a difficult subject on which to offer definitive advice. What I've described here is the type of tapering that has worked for me over the years; however, please don't be afraid to experiment with different approaches – it's the only way you're going to find out what best suits you.

So, with your training approach sorted and your programme working well for you, the next consideration is how to plan the race itself…

race day strategy

The perfect time to develop your race plan is during your taper training, when you've cut yourself a bit of slack. This is the moment for a reality check: what was your original goal? Have you done the training to support it?

Did you notice any indicators during the races you included as part of your training that you can carry over to improve your race day performance? Any strengths that you can profitably use, or weaknesses you need to work on trying to eliminate? What type and frequency of hydration and fuelling worked best for you in training?

Look back through the evidence in your training diary and calculate the splits you'll need to run to achieve your target time. Generally speaking, having tapered your training and hydrated and fuelled properly, together with the motivational lift you'll get from just participating in the event and the support of the crowds who come to spectate, you'll almost certainly run faster than you did in training. As long as you proceed at a controlled pace and don't make the fatal error of going out too quickly, you'll be fine. You should aim to run your second half slightly faster than the first, giving you a strong and comfortable finish. Ideally, you'll have enough left in the tank to pick up the pace in the closing stages of the race and finish with a flourish to wow your friends and family who came to watch you!

Revisit the refuelling and rehydrating methods that worked for you in training. If you used a particular gel or sports drink that particularly suited you (check out what, if any, sports drink the organisers will be handing out at water stops), then make sure you have a reliable means of carrying it. Re-read 'Race day tips' on page 98.

Take some time to visualise key sections of your race. Relax and imagine yourself running quickly and strongly over tough parts of the course and see yourself finishing well, feeling great and achieving your goal. I like to look back through my training diaries and pick out good training workouts and runs to remind myself of how well I have prepared. During particularly challenging stages of the race, it can really help to think back on how you felt in previous good moments and concentrate on recreating that positive feeling.

Set out your primary aim: if it's a time goal, make sure you know your target split times – but stay fully in touch with how you're feeling. If you're way up on your target times but feel good and controlled, have the confidence to stick with it. However, be very honest with yourself here. I remember en route to setting the new marathon world record in London in 2003, I knew I was way ahead of record pace, but I felt confident, controlled and strong. I didn't want to set a limit on how fast I could go, rather I wanted to judge my effort to get the very best time out of myself that day. To do this, I had to be very in tune with how my body and energy levels felt.

If you have a position goal – to win the race, or to beat a specific rival – then you need to plan your race strategy so that it plays to your strengths. No matter how great you think it looks to see someone sit in among the leaders the whole way and then kick strongly at the end, if you know that, realistically, you are not super-fast at the end, then this tactic is a waste of time. Rather, plan to inject pace earlier, making it a tougher, more sustained run; or attack on hills or twisty sections if these are your strong points.

Whatever your race strategy, always make sure you go into the race looking forward to it. After the hard training, races are the rewarding, fun part. Some nerves on the day are good, as these demonstrate that the race is important to you – plus, adrenaline levels help boost performance. However, too many nerves drain you and make the whole experience stressful rather than fun. If you find nerves getting too much, remind yourself that it's fun, then relax and take time out by chilling with family, reading a book or watching a film to get your mind off the race a bit.

Good luck, have fun with the training – and, especially, enjoy the race!

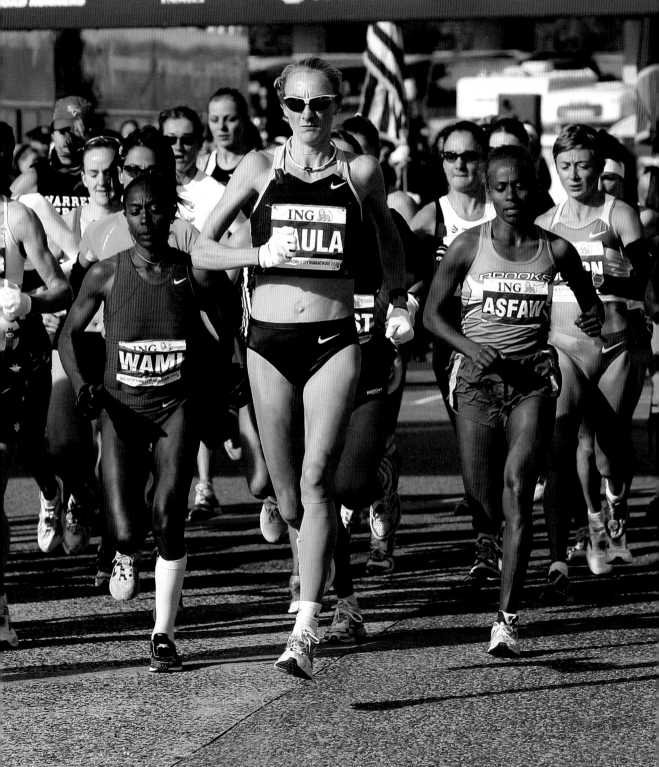

How to train for a fast 10K

notes

- I've made the rest day a Friday, but you can easily switch it to Monday or Wednesday if that works better for your family or work schedule.

- For your longer run on the weekend, look for a park with varied terrain or some other off-road route.

- I've included several track sessions; if you're not already a member of a running club, try to find one that you can join – training with others somehow feels easier and is definitely more fun. Sessions can be adapted to suit what the group is doing. If you don't have a track nearby, you can try pacing out and marking every 200m on grass or paths.

	monday	tuesday	wednesday
week 1	40 to 45-min easy/ steady run. Weights: Session A	2-mile warm-up. Stretches. 15 hill reps approx 200m long: run uphill, then jog down to recover. Do 2 sets of 7 and, after first set, take a slow walk down the hill. 2-mile jog.	35 to 40-min steady run. Weights: Session B. Include abs.
week 2	40 to 45-min easy/ steady run. Weights: Session A	2-mile warm-up and cool-down. Drills on road or grass: 8 x 3 mins hard effort (aim to run at target race pace or slightly faster). 90 sec to 2-min jog recovery.	35 to 40-min steady run. Weights: Session B. Include abs.
week 3	40 to 45-min easy/ steady run. Weights: Session A	20-mile warm-up and cool-down. Track session: 3–4 sets x 1,000m, 600m and 400m, with 200m jog recovery. Aim for 10K target race pace for the 1,000m reps, a bit faster for 600m and 400m.	35 to 40-min steady run. Weights: Session B. Include abs.
week 4	40 to 45-min easy/ steady run. Weights: Session A	2-mile warm-up and cool-down. Drills on road or grass: 8 x 4 mins of hard effort, with 90 sec to 2-min jog recovery between each.	35 to 40-min steady run. Weights: Session B. Include abs.
week 5	40 to 45-min easy/ steady run. Weights: Session A	2-mile warm-up and cool-down. Light drills on track (or marked path): 4 x 1,000m, 4 x 400m, 2 x 1,000m, 2 x 400m, with 200m jog recovery. Aim for 10K target race pace on the 1,000m reps, and slightly faster for 400m.	35 to 40-min steady run. Weights: Session B. Include abs.
week 6	40 to 45-min easy/ steady run. Weights: Session A	2-mile warm-up and cool-down. Drills on road or grass: 8 x 4 mins of hard effort, with 90 sec to 2-min jog recovery between each.	35 to 40-min steady run. Weights: Session B. Include abs.
week 7	40 to 45-min easy/ steady run. Weights: Session A	2-mile warm-up and down. Light drills: 4 sets of 1,000m, 600m, 400m reps (as before). 200m jog to recover between each.	35 to 40-min steady run. Weights: Session B. Include abs.
week 8	30-min easy run. Weights: Session A (light session)	2-mile warm-up and cool-down. Drills on a good path or grass: 8 to 10 x 2 mins of reps, controlled and feeling strong, 90-secs jog recovery in between.	30-min steady run. 3 to 4 x 80m strides. Core exercises.

1 mile = 1.6 km, 1.5 miles = 2.4 km, 2 miles = 3.25 km, 3 miles = 4.8 km, 4 miles = 6.5 km, 5 miles = 8 km, 6 miles = 9.5 km, 7 miles = 11.25 km

- I've also added more drills and strides before and after runs in order to keep the faster twitch muscles ticking over and to help your running form.

- The biggest change is the addition of weights and strength training from Chapter 3, Taking care of your body. Assuming you are already doing some work with weights, start with two weekly sessions (if you're not, then be sure to ease in more gradually) and, also, some core strength sessions. The third session is totally optional.

- I know I've said this before several times in this book, but it can never be said often enough: always, unfailingly, stretch after you've finished training. This is essential preventative work to help guard against injury.

thursday	friday	saturday	sunday
1.5-mile warm-up and cool-down. Drills: Tempo introduction: 3-mile tempo run. 1-mile jog. 2-mile tempo run.	Rest day: Some core exercises and an optional Session C weights programme.	1-mile warm-up and cool-down. 35 mins of fartlek. Varying-length reps from 20 secs to 2 mins. Easy runs to recover between reps.	8 to 10-mile steady off-road run. Core exercises.
1-mile warm-up and cool-down. 5-mile tempo run.	Rest day: Some core exercises and an optional Session C weights programme.	1-mile warm-up and cool-down. Drills: 35 mins of fartlek.	8 to 10-mile steady off-road run. Core exercises.
1-mile warm-up and cool-down. Sustained fartlek tempo run: 2 miles slightly above tempo pace (HR: 85–90% of max), 1-mile steady and 2 miles faster to finish.	Rest day: Some core exercises and an optional Session C weights programme.	1-mile warm-up and cool-down. Drills: 40 mins of fartlek.	8 to 10-mile steady off-road run. Core exercises.
1-mile warm-up and cool-down. 6-mile tempo run.	Rest day: Some core exercises and an optional Session C weights programme.	1-mile warm-up and cool-down. Drills: 40 mins of fartlek.	8 to 10-mile steady off-road run. Core exercises.
1-mile warm-up and cool-down. 3 x 2 miles at a good pace: aim to get heart rate up to 90–95% of max. 2 to 3 mins easy jog in between.	Rest day: Some core exercises and an optional Session C weights programme.	1-mile warm-up and cool-down. Drills: 40 mins of fartlek.	9 to 10-mile off-road run. Core exercises.
1-mile warm-up and cool down. 6-mile tempo run.	Rest day: Some core exercises and an optional Session C weights programme.	1-mile warm-up and cool-down. Drills: 40 mins of fartlek.	10-mile off-road run. Core exercises.
1-mile warm-up and cool-down. 5-mile tempo run.	Rest day: Some core exercises and an optional Session C weights programme.	1-mile warm-up and cool-down. Drills. 35 mins of fartlek.	8-mile off-road run. Core exercises.
Option: Rest day or 20-min easy run. Drills: 3 to 5 x 80m–100m strides, with walk-back recovery.	Rest day if you ran yesterday. Otherwise do yesterday's 20-min easy run, drills and strides today.	Rest day.	**RACE DAY**

8 miles = 12.9 km, 9 miles = 14.5 km, 10 miles = 16 km

How to train for a fast half-marathon

• I've worked on the assumption that you have already followed a programme of some sort for previous half-marathons that you've run.

• I've made Friday the rest day, but still included some core work. However, this can easily be swapped with the Wednesday or even the Monday, if you prefer. If you're racing, switch it back to the day before.

• Stretching is a must before and after each and every run.

	monday	tuesday	wednesday
week 1	40-min easy run. Gym weights programme: Session A. Don't forget the abs!	2-mile warm-up. 8 x 3-min hard runs (try to get HR above 80%). 2-min slow jog recovery. 2-mile cool-down.	45-min steady/ easy run. Gym weights programme: Session B.
week 2	40-min easy run. Gym weights programme: Session A.	2-mile warm-up. 9 x 3-min hard runs (try to get HR above 80%). 2-min slow jog recovery. 2-mile cool-down.	8-mile easy run Gym weights programme: Session B.
week 3	45-min easy run. Gym weights programme: Session A.	2-mile warm-up. 6 x 5-min hard runs. 2 to 3-min slow jog recovery. 2-mile cool-down.	8-mile easy run Gym weights programme: Session B.
week 4	45-min easy run. Gym weights programme: Session A.	2-mile warm-up. 10 x 3-min hard runs. 2-min jog recovery. **Or**: on a track, 4 sets x 1,000m, 800m, 600m reps, with 200m jog between reps. 2-mile cool-down.	8-mile easy run Gym weights programme: Session B.
week 5	45-min easy run. Gym weights programme: Session A.	2-mile warm-up. 5 x 6-min hard effort. 2-min slow jog in between. 2-mile cool-down.	8-mile easy run. Gym weights programme: Session B.
week 6	45-min easy run Gym weights programme: Session A.	2-mile warm-up. **Either** track: 6 x 800m, 6 x 400m hard effort, 200m jog in between. 2-mile cool-down. **Or**: 3 sets x 4-min, 3-min, 2-min hard effort on grass or road with 2-min jog recovery. (Warm-up and cool-down as before.)	8-mile easy run. Gym weights programme: Session B.
week 7	45-min easy run Gym weights programme: Session A.	2-mile warm-up. 5 x 6-min hard runs. 2-minute jog recovery. 2-mile cool-down.	8-mile easy run. Gym weights programme: Session B.
week 8	45-min easy run. Gym weights programme: Session A.	2-mile warm-up. **Either** track: 8 x 1,000m reps, with 200m jog in between. **Or**: on grass or road, 8 x 4-min hard effort. 2-min jog recovery. 2-mile cool-down.	9-mile easy run. Gym weights programme: Session B.
week 9	45-min easy run. Gym weights programme: Session A.	2-mile warm-up. Mixed tempo run: 2 miles faster than target race pace, 1 mile slower, 2 miles faster. 2-mile cool-down.	8-mile easy run. Gym weights programme: Session B.
week 10	45-min easy run. Gym weights programme: Session A.	2-mile warm-up. 6 x 6-min hard effort on road, with 2-min jog recovery. 2-mile cool-down.	8 to 9-mile easy run. Gym weights programme: Session B.
week 11	45-min easy run. Gym weights programme: Session A.	2-mile warm-up. **Either**: track: 9 x 1,000m hard effort at 10K race pace, with 200m jog recovery. **Or**: 10 x 3-min hard runs on grass or road, with 90-second jog recovery. 2-mile cool-down.	8-mile easy run. Gym weights programme: Session B.
week 12	Rest or 3 to 4-mile easy run. Core strength and conditioning at home.	2-mile warm-up. 8 x 2-min controlled effort at 10K race pace, with 90-sec jog recovery. 2-mile cool-down.	Rest if you ran Monday. **Or**: 3 to 4-mile easy run. Core strength exercises.

1 mile = 1.6 km, 1.5 miles = 2.4 km, 2 miles = 3.25 km, 3 miles = 4.8 km, 4 miles = 6.5 km, 5 miles = 8 km, 6 miles = 9.5 km, 7 miles = 11.25 km

Tip: For the Saturday fartlek session, run with friends and take turns picking the length of pace pick-ups. Or get a friend/kids to come on a bike and blow a whistle for each change of pace.
Tip: Join a running club – it's more fun running, especially if you're doing track sessions. And by all means change these to something similar to the group sessions at the club.
Tip: Try to slightly improve your tempo run each time.
Tip: Get a weekly massage, even if it's just from your other half!
Tip: Experiment with 10 minutes in a cold/ice water bath

thursday	friday	saturday	sunday
1-mile jog warm-up. 6-mile tempo run. 1-mile jog cool-down.	Rest day. Core strength exercises and stretches.	2-mile jog. Stretches. On a 200–250m hill, run: 2 sets x 7 hills, concentrating on good form. Jog down recovery and walk between sets.1–2-mile jog.	10 to 12-mile steady run, off-road if possible. Practise drinking during.
1-mile jog warm-up. 6.5-mile tempo run. 1-mile jog cool-down.	Rest day. Core strength exercises and stretches.	1.5-mile jog. Stretches. 40 mins of fartlek: set off at easy pace, picking it up to faster for stretches varying from 20 secs–2 mins. Slow to easy pace to recover, then go again. 2-mile jog.	12-mile steady run, off-road if possible. Practise drinking during.
1-mile jog warm-up. 6.5-mile tempo run. 1-mile jog cool-down.	Rest day. Core strength exercises and stretches.	2-mile jog. Stretches. On a 200–250m hill, run: 15 hills, concentrating on good form. Jog down recovery. 2-mile jog.	12-mile steady run, off-road if possible. Practise drinking during.
1-mile warm-up. 7-mile tempo run. 1-mile cool-down.	Rest day. Core strength exercises and stretches.	1-mile jog. Stretches. 45 mins fartlek as per week 2. 1-mile jog.	13-mile steady run, off-road if possible. Practise drinking during.
1-mile warm-up. 7-mile tempo run. 1-mile cool-down.	Rest day. Core strength exercises and stretches.	2-mile jog. Stretches. On a 200–250m hill, run: 15 hills, concentrating on good form. Jog down recovery. 2-mile jog.	14-mile steady run, off-road if possible. Practise drinking during.
1.5-mile warm-up. If racing on Sat: 3 to 4-mile controlled tempo run (pace as per longer tempo run). If not racing: 6.5-mile tempo run. 1.5-mile cool-down.	Rest day. Core strength exercises and stretches.	Race: 5-mile or 10K race. Good warm-up and cool-down. **Or:** 1-mile warm-up. Stretches. 45 mins of fartlek. 1-mile cool-down.	14-mile steady run, off-road if possible. Practise drinking during.
2-mile jog. Sustained tempo fartlek: 2 miles at faster than race pace; 1 mile slower than race pace; 2 miles faster than race pace; 1 mile a bit slower; 1 mile faster to finish. 1-mile easy jog.	Rest day. Core strength exercises and stretches.	2-mile jog. Stretches. On a 200–250m hill, run: 15 hills, concentrating on good form. Jog down recovery. 2-mile jog.	15-mile steady run, off-road if possible. Practise drinking during.
1-mile jog. 7-mile tempo run. 1-mile jog.	Rest day. Core strength exercises and stretches.	1-mile jog. Stretching. 50 mins of fartlek. 1-mile jog	13-mile steady run, off-road if possible. Practise drinking during.
1-2-mile jog. 3 to 4 good-paced 100m strides (walk back). 5 x 3-min sustained runs at 70-80% of max HR, feeling fast but comfortable, with 90-sec jog recovery. 1-2-mile jog.	Rest day. **Or:** Optional 20-min easy jog. Core strength exercises and stretches.	Rest day.	10K race. Warm up well beforehand and jog a mile slowly afterwards. (Run a little faster than the last race.)
1-mile warm-up. 7-8-mile tempo run. 1-mile cool-down.	Rest day. Core strength exercises and stretches.	1-mile jog. Stretches. 45–50 mins of fartlek. 1-mile jog.	13 to 14-mile steady run, off-road if possible. Practise drinking during.
1-mile warm-up. 6-mile tempo run. 3-4 x 100m strides with walk back recovery. 1.5-mile cool-down.	Rest day. Core strength exercises and stretches.	2-mile jog. Stretches. On a 200–250m hill, run: 15 reps, concentrating on good form. Jog down recovery. 2-mile jog.	10-mile steady/easy run, off-road if possible. Practise drinking during.
6-mile easy run.	Rest. **Or:** Optional 3-mile easy run. Some light core strength exercises and stretching.	Rest day.	**HALF-MARATHON RACE DAY**

8 miles = 12.9 km, 9 miles = 14.5 km, 10 miles = 16 km, 11 miles = 17.7 km, 12 miles = 19.3 km, 13 miles = 21 km, 14 miles = 22.5 km, 15 miles = 24 km

How to train for a fast marathon

	monday	tuesday	wednesday
week 1	45-min easy/steady run. Gym weights programme: Session A.	2-mile warm-up. On road or 'good' grass: 6–8 x 3-min reps (aim for your 10K race pace), with 90 sec to 2-min jog recovery in between. 2-mile cool-down.	8 to 10-mile steady/easy run. Gym weights programme: Session B.
week 2	50-min easy/steady run. Gym weights programme: Session A. Include core exercises.	2-mile warm-up. On road or grass: 5-6 x 5-min reps. 2-min jog recovery. 2-mile cool-down.	8 to 10-mile steady/easy run. Gym weights programme: Session B.
week 3	50-min easy/steady run. Gym weights programme: Session A. Include core exercises.	2-mile warm-up. **Option**: Track session (10K race pace): 2x1000m, 2x400m (recovery), 2x1000m, 2x400m, 2x1000m. 200m jog recovery between reps. **Or**: Road/grass: 8 x 3-min reps, 90-sec jog recovery. 2-mile cool-down.	8 to 10-mile steady/easy run. Gym weights programme: Session B.
week 4	50-min easy/steady run. Gym weights programme: Session A. Include core exercises.	2-mile warm-up. On road or grass: 5 x 6-min reps at about 85% max HR, with 2-min jog recovery between each. 2-mile jog cool-down.	10-mile steady/easy run. Gym weights programme: Session B.
week 5	50-min easy/steady run. Gym weights programme: Session A. Include core exercises.	2-mile warm-up. **Option**: Track session: 3–4 sets of 1,200m and 800m reps, with 200m-jog recovery between reps. **Or**: On road or grass: 9 x 3-min reps, with 90-sec jog recovery. 2-mile cool-down.	10-mile steady/easy run. Gym weights programme: Session B.
week 6	50-min easy/steady run. Gym weights programme: Session A. Include core exercises.	2-mile warm-up. 5 x 6-min hard efforts, with 2-min jog recovery between each. 2-mile cool-down.	8-mile steady/easy run. Gym weights programme: Session B (go light if racing this weekend).
week 7	50-min easy/steady run. Gym weights programme: Session A. Include core exercises.	2-mile warm-up. If racing: 6 to 8 x 3-min efforts, with 90-sec jog recovery. If not racing: 8–10 reps. **Or**: Track session: 4 x 1,000m, 600m, 400m, with 200m-jog recovery between reps. 2-mile cool-down.	8-mile steady/easy run. Gym weights programme: Session B (go light if racing).
week 8	50-min easy/steady run. Gym weights programme: Session A. Include core exercises.	2-mile warm-up. 5 x 6-min hard efforts, 2-min jog recovery between each. 2-mile cool-down.	10-mile steady/easy run. Gym weights programme: Session B.
week 9	50-min easy/steady run. Gym weights programme: Session A. Include core exercises.	2-mile warm-up. On road or 'good' grass: 2-min, 3-min, 4-min, 5-min, 6-min, 5-min, 4-min and 3-min efforts, with 90-sec jog recovery in between. 2-mile cool-down.	10-mile steady/easy run. Gym weights programme: Session B.
week 10	50-min easy/steady run. Gym weights programme: Session A. Include core exercises.	2-mile warm-up. On road: 5-6 x 1 mile, 2-min jog recovery in between. 2-mile cool-down.	10-mile steady/easy run. Gym weights programme: Session B.
week 11	40-45-min easy/steady run. Gym weights programme: Session A. Include core exercises.	2-mile warm-up. If racing this w/e: 8–10 x 2-min reps, 90-sec jog recovery. If not: **Either**: On road/grass: 8–10 x 3-min efforts, 90-sec jog recovery. **Or**: track: 6–8 x 1000m, with 200m jog recovery. 2-mile cool-down.	10-mile steady/easy run (8 miles if racing). Gym weights programme: Session B (skip it if racing this week).
week 12	45-min easy/steady run. Gym weights programme: Session A. Include core exercises.	2-mile warm-up. If racing this w/e: 8–10 x 2-min reps, 90-sec jog recovery. If not racing: **Either**: 8–10 x 3-min efforts, 90-sec jog recovery. **Or**: Track: 6–8 x 1,000m, with 200m-jog recovery. 2-mile cool-down.	10-mile steady/easy run (8 miles if racing). Gym weights programme: Session B (skip it if racing this week).
week 13	50-min easy/steady run. Gym weights programme: Session A. Include core exercises.	2-mile warm-up. On road or grass: 5 x 6-min efforts, 2-min jog recovery between each. 2-mile cool-down.	10 to 12-mile steady/easy run. Gym weights programme: Session B.
week 14	50-min easy/steady run. Core exercises. Gentle gym weights programme: Session A (light weights only).	2-mile warm-up. **Either**: Track: 6–8 x 1,000m, with 200m-jog recovery. **Or**: On road/grass: 8 x 3 min 30 sec efforts, with 90-sec jog recovery.	9-mile steady/easy run. Core exercises.
week 15	40-min steady run. Core exercises.	2-mile warm-up. On road: 5 x 4–5-min efforts. 2-min jog recovery between each. (Test race-day shoes and kit.) 1-mile cool-down.	7-mile steady/easy run. Core exercises.
week 16	Rest day. Easy session of core exercises.	6-mile easy run. 4 x 100m strides.	5-mile easy run. 4 x 100m strides.

1 mile = 1.6 km, 1.5 miles = 2.4 km, 2 miles = 3.25 km, 3 miles = 4.8 km, 4 miles = 6.5 km, 5 miles = 8 km, 6 miles = 9.5 km, 7 miles = 11.25 km, 8 miles = 12.9 km, 9 miles = 14.5 km, 10 miles = 16 km, 11 miles = 17.7 km, 12 miles = 19.3 km, 13 miles = 21 km, 14 miles = 22.5 km, 15 miles = 24 km, 16 miles = 25.7 km
17 miles = 27.3 km, 18 miles = 29 km, 19 miles = 30.5 km, 20 miles = 32 km, 21 miles = 34 km, 22 miles = 35.5 km, 23 miles = 37 km

thursday	friday	saturday	sunday
2-mile warm-up. 6-mile tempo run. 2-mile cool-down.	Rest day. Core exercises at home.	8 to 10-mile run at a good pace, including some hills. **Optional**: Gym weights programme: (light weights) Session C.	14-mile run off-road if possible. Practise drinking and refuelling on the run.
1.5-mile warm-up. 7-mile tempo run. 2-mile cool-down.	Rest day. Core exercises.	2-mile warm-up. 35 to 40-min reps up a 200–300m hill, focusing on good form and knee lift. Jog down recovery. 2-mile cool-down. **Optional**: Gym weights programme: (light weights) Session C.	15-mile run off-road if possible. Practise drinking and refuelling on the run.
1.5-mile warm-up. 8-mile tempo run. 1.5-mile cool-down.	Rest day. Core exercises.	2-mile warm-up. 40 mins of fartlek, pick up the pace for varying lengths from 20 secs to 3 mins. Jog to recover. 1-mile cool-down. **Optional**: Gym weights programme: (light weights) Session C.	17-mile run off-road if possible. Practise drinking and refuelling on the run.
1.5-mile warm-up. 9-mile tempo run. 1-mile cool-down.	Rest day. Core exercises.	2-mile warm-up. 45 mins of fartlek. 2-mile cool-down. **Optional**: Gym weights programme: (light weights) Session C.	18-mile run off-road if possible. Practise drinking and refuelling on the run.
1.5-mile warm-up. 9-mile tempo run. 1-mile cool-down.	Rest day. Core exercises.	2-mile warm-up. 45 mins of fartlek, with half a mile to 1-mile surges. Recovery miles at a steadier pace. 1-mile cool-down. **Optional**: Gym weights programme: (light weights) Session C	16 to 18-mile run off-road if possible (depending when/if racing). Practise drinking and refuelling.
2-mile warm-up. Light session of 8 x 1-min controlled pace (fast, not hard), with 90-sec jog in between. 2-mile cool-down.	Rest day. Core exercises.	Rest day, if racing tomorrow. **Or**: 2-mile warm-up. 45 mins of fartlek, including some hills. 1-mile cool-down.	10K race. **Or**: 16-mile run off-road if possible. Practise drinking and refuelling.
1.5-mile warm-up. 10-mile tempo run. **Or**: Same session as last week, if racing this weekend. 1.5-mile cool-down.	Rest day. Core exercises.	Rest day, if racing tomorrow. **Or**: 2-mile warm-up. 45 mins fartlek, including some hills. 1-mile cool-down. If not racing: Gym weights programme: (light weights) Session C.	10K race, if you didn't race last weekend. **Or**: 18-mile run off-road if possible. Practise drinking and refuelling.
1.5-mile warm-up. 9-mile tempo run. 5 x 6-min efforts. 8-min jog recovery. 1.5-mile cool-down.	Rest day. Core exercises.	2-mile warm-up. 50 mins of fartlek. 2-mile cool-down. **Option**: Gym (light) weights programme: Session C.	21-mile run off-road if possible. Practise drinking and refuelling.
1.5-mile warm-up. 10-mile tempo run. 1.5-mile cool-down.	Rest Day. Core exercises.	2-mile warm-up. 50 mins of fartlek. 1-mile cool-down. **Optional**: Gym (light) weights programme: Session C.	23-mile run off-road if possible. Practise drinking and refuelling.
1.5-mile warm-up. 10-mile tempo run. 1.5-mile cool-down.	Rest day. Core exercises.	2-mile warm-up. Hill reps: 40 mins of reps on a 250–300m hill. Jog-down recovery. 2-mile cool-down. **Optional**: Gym weights programme: (light weights) Session C.	22-mile run off-road if possible. Practise drinking and refuelling.
If racing this week, 40-min steady/easy run. If not racing: good warm-up and cool-down. 8-mile tempo run.	Rest day. Core exercises.	Rest, if racing. **Or**: 2-mile warm-up. 45 mins of fartlek. 1-mile cool-down.	Half-marathon race. **Or**: 18 to 20-mile run off-road if possible. Practise drinking and refuelling.
If racing this week, 40-min steady/easy run. Strides. If not racing: warm-up and cool-down. 8 to 10-mile tempo run.	Rest day. Core exercises.	Rest, if racing. **Or**: 2-mile warm-up. 50 mins of fartlek. 1-mile cool-down.	Half-marathon race. **Or**: 22-mile run, off-road if possible. Practise drinking and refuelling.
1.5-mile warm-up. 10-mile tempo run. 1.5-mile cool-down.	Rest day. Core exercises.	2-mile warm-up. 40 mins hill reps. Jog-down recovery between each. 1-mile cool-down.	18 to 20-mile run off-road if possible. Practise drinking and refuelling.
1.5-mile warm-up. 7-mile tempo run. 1.5-mile cool-down.	Rest day. Core exercises.	1.5-mile warm-up. 40–45 mins of fartlek. 1.5-mile cool-down.	15-mile run off-road if possible. Practise drinking and refuelling.
1.5-mile warm-up. 5-mile tempo run (controlled and feeling good). 1.5-mile cool-down.	Rest day. Core exercises.	2-mile warm-up. 35 mins of fartlek. 1-mile jog cool-down.	10-mile run (12 miles max), off-road if possible. Practise drinking and refuelling.
3-mile jog. 4 x 100m strides. **Option**: Swap this with tomorrow's rest day.	Rest day. Core exercises.	Rest day.	**MARATHON RACE DAY**

7 mind games

The importance of your mind in determining the outcome of a race is critical. Learn to lift yourself to the next level by increasing your mental strength.

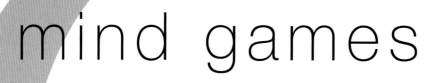

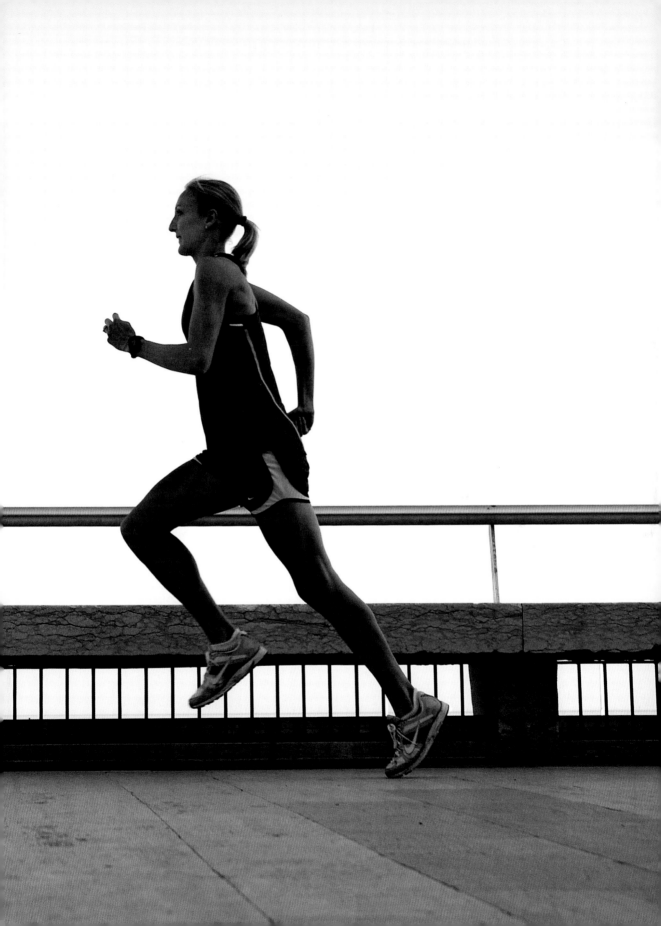

gaining an edge

When you first take up running, what gets you out the door is sheer enjoyment. It's this that motivates you to complete your first race (and fans the desire to target your second and third…) and gives you the immense satisfaction of putting a hard-earned tick next to 'goal' in your training diary.

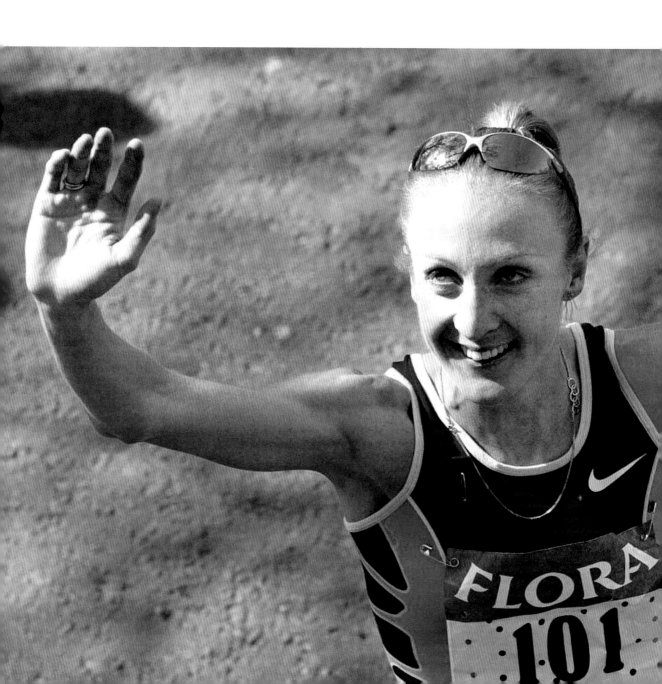

As you become more experienced and begin to get an idea of your potential, you may start wondering whether it might be worth complementing your physical training with exercises to strengthen your mind. This is often prompted by something you've read or through talking to experienced runners who use it as a means of gaining a competitive edge. They do this by learning how to control their performance through developing consistency in training and racing. They also spend time working at sharpening their ability to concentrate.

In long distance events, the importance of your state of mind in determining the outcome of a race can't be overestimated. Exploring ways of lifting yourself to the next level by increasing your mental strength and, in the process, greatly building your confidence, will pay dividends – not only in terms of your running performance, but in life in general, as well.

In this chapter, I'll be taking a look at techniques that you may find helpful.

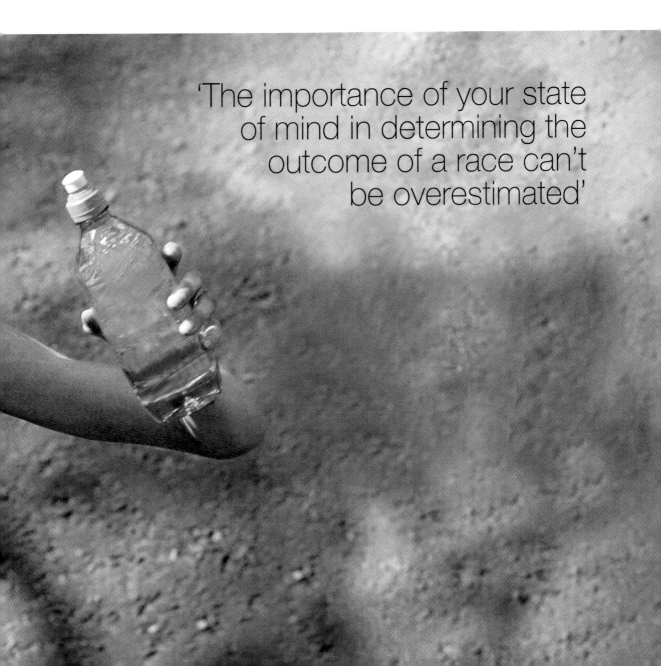

'The importance of your state of mind in determining the outcome of a race can't be overestimated'

optimise your performance

You'll read a lot about cognitive strategies in sport, but far from focusing on the race at hand, less experienced distance runners try to distract themselves with thoughts that take their mind off their tiredness. This can mean, however, that they are less aware of how their bodies are performing.

On the other hand, more experienced runners do the opposite: they try to stay in the moment, focusing on performing as effortlessly as possible. They do everything they can to conserve energy and maintain efficiency, running lightly on their feet rather than pounding the ground hard, and constantly riffling through a checklist of how their body is coping. They also focus on their weaker areas – the places where they know fatigue tends to set in first. This could mean adjusting their shoulders to keep the upper body loose; identifying other areas of muscle tension (or, indeed, laziness) and consciously working on relaxing them or stimulating them. Examples might be: unclenching hands and fingers; monitoring foot strike and stride pattern; firing up the glutes properly; ensuring that the arms are swinging forwards and backwards, rather than from side to side; maintaining awareness of hydration levels; observing breathing patterns; working out split times; watching competitors and – in my case – counting in my head to determine where I am within each mile.

This is something that I started doing a long time ago as a means of focusing on where I was within each grass/road rep that was run to time, rather than marked distance. I found it helped me to judge and pace myself. As I moved to road races, I learned that breaking each mile down worked well for me. For a half or full marathon pace, counting three times to 100 roughly equates to a mile: this technique helps me focus on where I am within each mile of the race and has become my technique for anchoring my concentration. I use it to truly stay in the moment.

So, it's pretty clear that maintaining good form optimises running efficiency and performance. This is why experienced runners try out psychological strategies during higher intensity sessions such as hills and intervals, when fatigue can sometimes threaten to overwhelm and weaken their technique. It's for this reason that in the training programmes at the end of Chapters 5 and 6 I sometimes refer to maintaining good form in hill training. If you can run with technical precision under duress, you'll have no difficulty maintaining good form the rest of the time and in races.

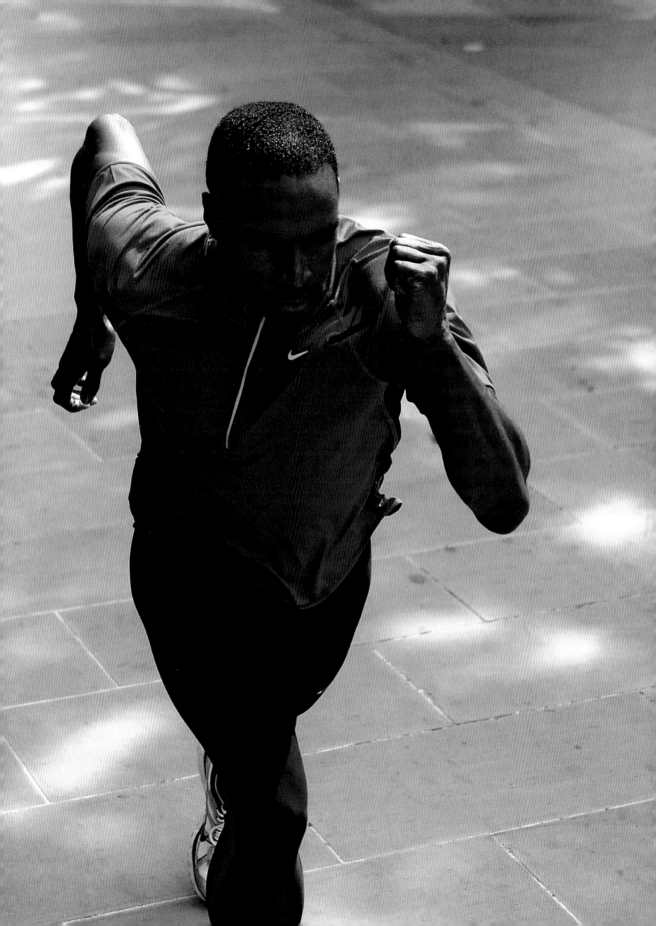

in the zone

No chapter on the mental aspect of training and competing would be complete without the much-discussed state commonly known as 'flow' or, as many athletes now describe it: being 'in the zone'.

This state of mind comes about when you are so utterly absorbed in the task at hand that you feel as though you're in a trance-like state, completely in control and effortlessly performing to the exclusion of all external distractions.

You'll probably have observed this happening in quite a few sports – those moments during a tennis match, for instance, when a player suddenly seems invincible: his limbs move smoothly and flawlessly as perfect, almost robotic extensions of his brain; his senses are in a heightened yet relaxed state of alertness, seizing opportunities as they present themselves and making impossible shots somehow look easy. What he's experiencing, says renowned Hungarian psychologist Mihaly Csikszentmihalyi, the man who popularised the term, is 'flow'. Before the 1990 publication of Csikszentmihalyi's seminal work on the subject, no such word existed to describe this state of mind so effectively. Today, however, you hear it from world leaders, business management gurus and top-class sportsmen and women alike.

Csikszentmihalyi was fascinated by the whole subject of enjoyment. He used his post-doctoral research opportunity to study what made artists contented and fulfilled. Then he broadened the programme to include thousands of other people from different walks of life all over the world. It was from these research subjects that he first heard the term 'flow' being used as a metaphor to explain how they were feeling. Several described their experience as a feeling of being 'carried away by a current, everything moving smoothly, without effort'. From the collation of these accounts, he distilled his findings into a list of conditions, one or more of which needed to be present in order for the participant to experience 'flow'. They boiled down to seven conditions:

- challenging activities requiring skill and effort;
- a clearly defined goal on which participants could focus their attention;
- deep concentration;
- immediate feedback that told them that their effort had produced a positive result, and enabled them to move on to the next level of the task;
- a sense of effortless control;
- total absence of self-consciousness, as though the boundaries between the self and the task had melted away, allowing the two to merge into one seamless entity;
- the sensation of time standing still, the seconds and hours rushing past unnoticed.

My sharpest and possibly most memorable experience of being in the 'zone' was during the World Cross Country Championships in Ostend in 2001, where I won the senior long race for the first time. That day, I felt surreally cool and in control. It was almost as though I knew what would happen before it did. A calm voice in my head seemed to tell me exactly what moves to make and when. I just knew I would win that race.

Maintaining a state of flow throughout an entire marathon is a tall order. Most of us bounce between distracting ourselves with visions of palm-fringed beaches and steering our thoughts back to concerns directly related to the race. Yet there's no doubt that when the physical training is done, it's the psychological factors that most affect our performance and turn the big events into self-fulfilling prophecies, good or bad. Try looking back and comparing a race or training session where you felt happy and in control with another where you felt stressed. See what I mean? Consistent practice of mental skills, plus focusing your mind on recreating that happy relaxed feeling, can make the difference between having a good day and an off day.

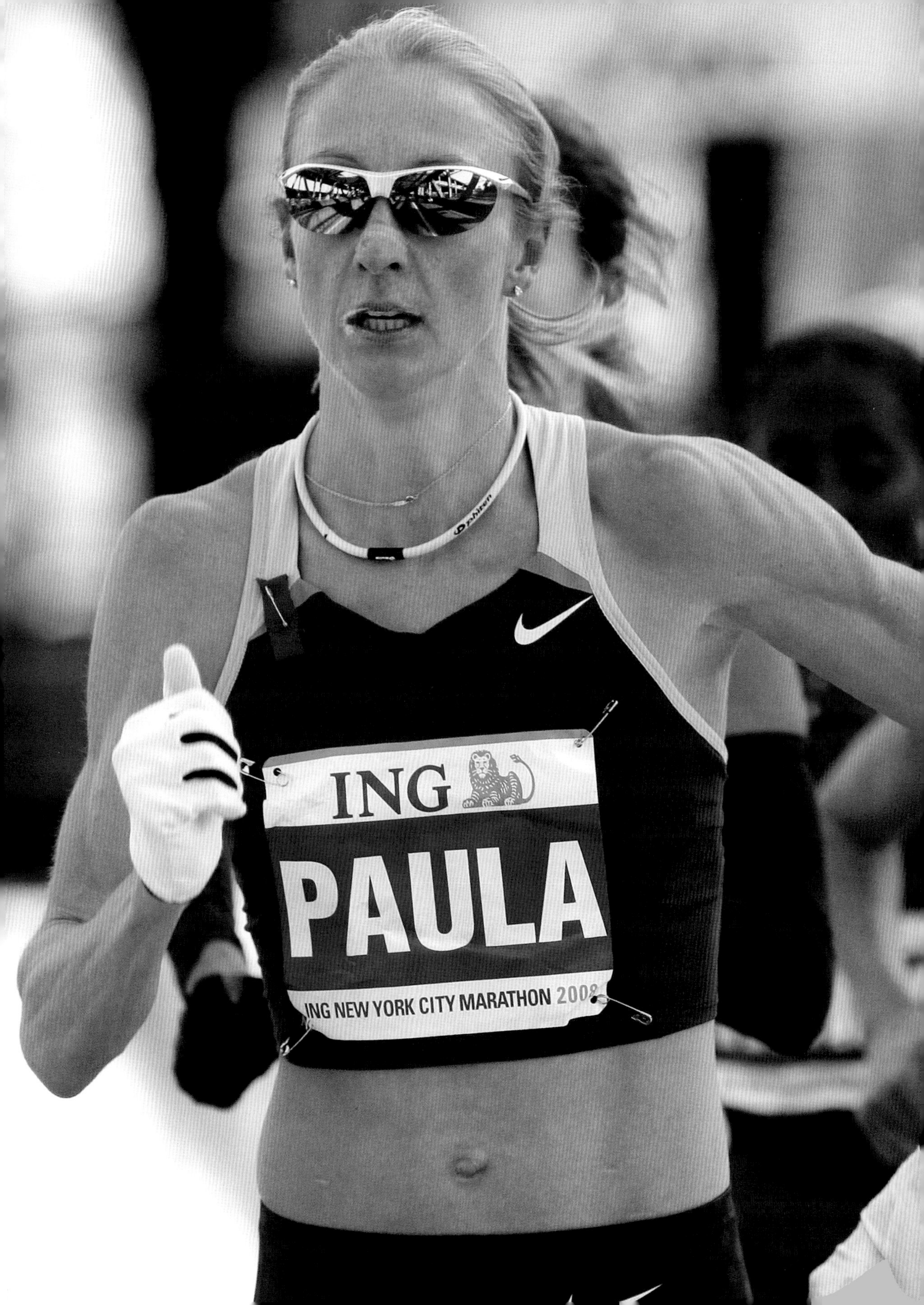
ING
PAULA
ING NEW YORK CITY MARATHON 2008

how do you 'flow'?

1 Prepare thoroughly

The crucial foundation stone is solid preparation. By this, I mean preparing for your key training sessions just as you would prepare for a race. Set your objectives and a game plan for the session; map out your splits and keep an eye on your times; run through your performance checklist in your mind, staying relaxed and making physical adjustments as necessary. This will help bring your mind back to the present when your concentration goes walkabout.

2 Relax

It's worth emphasising this as a point in its own right: the more relaxed you are, the more chance you'll have of getting into a state of flow. Keep your shoulders down and remind yourself to smile – smiling (and yawning) are useful stress-relievers.

3 Visualise success

Use the power of your imagination to conjure up the feeling of achieving your goal. Try to bring all your senses to the task: imagine crossing the line at the end of the race; visualise the time on the clock at the finish; smell the menthol from the muscle ointment around you; hear the cheers from the spectators; feel the texture of the medal and the ribbon around your neck; bask in the congratulations from your friends and family.

Remember what I said about goal-setting in Chapter 1? The unconscious mind doesn't differentiate between a real experience and a vividly imagined one, so rehearsing a positive outcome brings you closer to achieving it. This is a major plank in the mind training done by world-class athletes of all types. I make a point of always visiting the finishing straight of big races in the days beforehand just so that I can visualise and judge my finish correctly.

4 Talk to yourself

This complements creative visualisation. Psychologists estimate that we conduct a steady stream of internal conversation with ourselves amounting to around 300 words a minute. Just imagine if you could harness this subconscious stream of chatter and turn a load of old boring reminders such as 'Put the bins out in the morning' into an opportunity for reprogramming yourself and giving yourself a good pep talk when you need it. Well, you can.

We know from the many years of research that have been invested in exploring this complex subject that negative thoughts produce negative emotions; they, in turn, lead to negative outcomes. But the reverse is equally true: positive feelings lead to high self-belief, confidence and positive results.

So, it's pretty obvious: start practising mind games now and steal ahead of your closest competitors. When you're competing against runners who have similar physical potential to yourself, it's very often mental muscle that gives you the power to edge ahead of them.

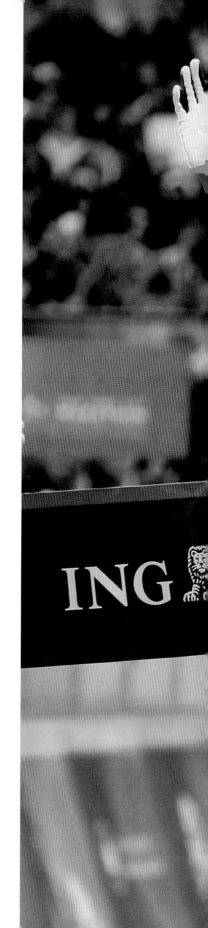

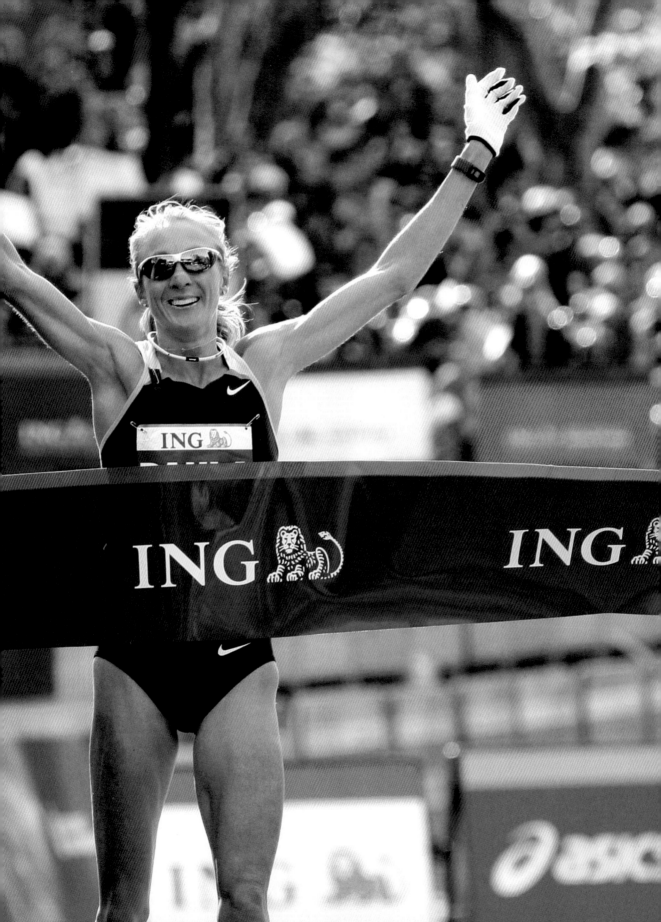

become your own motivator

Try these steps towards learning to motivate yourself:

- Write down a brief affirmation that describes you, stating it in the present. For example: 'I've put in the hard work and I'm ready to take on the challenge'; 'I'm supremely capable of running x miles in y minutes'; 'I'm in great shape and fully prepared for such-and-such a race'. Use words that express it emphatically and in the positive.
- Now say it out loud. This is the key: when you give voice to something, what was previously a thought that just blended in with the rest of the subconscious chatter in your mind now stands apart from it as a bold, spoken statement that you have witnessed yourself saying aloud. Repeat it 10–20 times and give it your full attention. Look yourself in the eye in the mirror as you say it.
- Next, choose specific words that describe aspects of the checklist that you'll be going through when you're training and racing. These are called 'trigger words'; say these to yourself while you're running. For instance, 'loose', 'smooth', 'easy', 'steady', 'shoulders down', 'relaxed arms' (come up with ones that suit you) that you instantly associate with good technique and strategy.
- Lastly, think exclusively about previous positive experiences – don't allow anything that historically had a negative outcome to enter your mind.

Every night before you go to bed, clear your brain and talk to yourself, defining and articulating your aims and objectives. Then visualise them happening before you drift off to sleep.

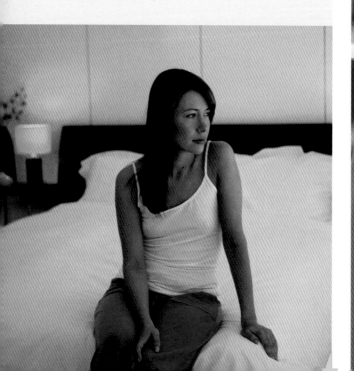

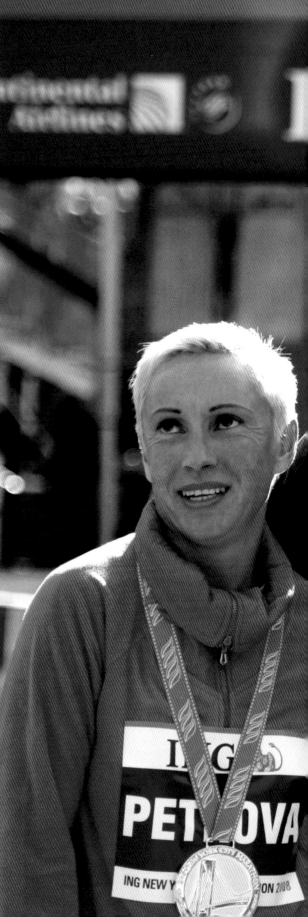

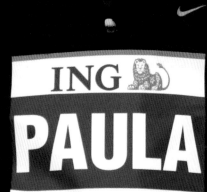

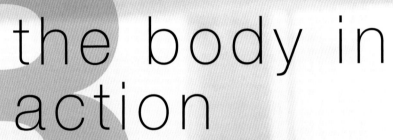

the body in action

8

Understanding what makes your body tick
and learning how to look after it is the key
to unlocking your potential.

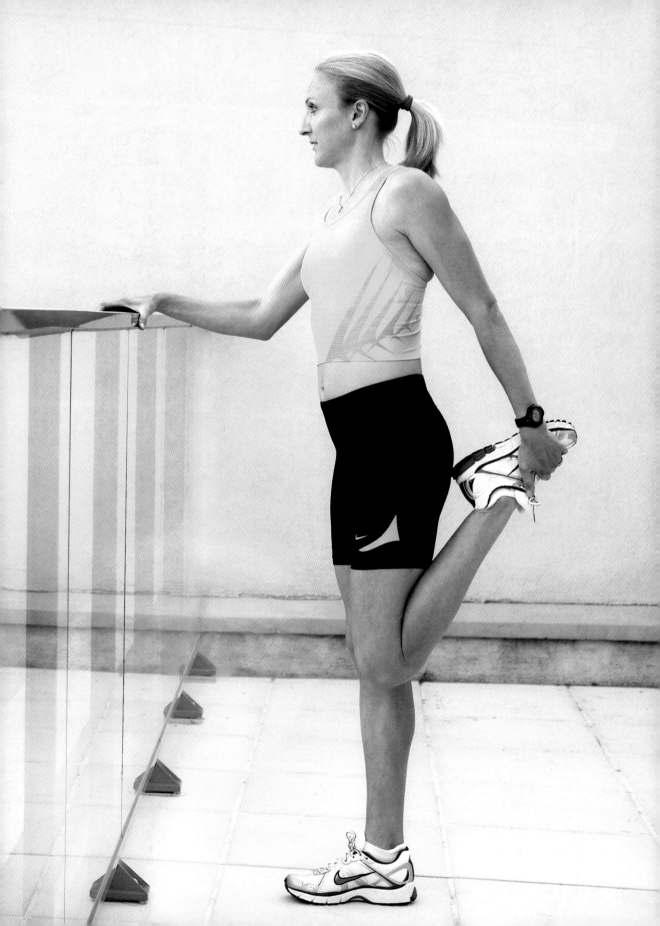

knowledge is power

The first time we run a long-distance race, the big question on everyone's lips is: how will my body behave? I say 'behave' rather than 'perform' because, thanks to the hours spent training to cover distances we never dreamt we'd be capable of running, we know how we can perform.

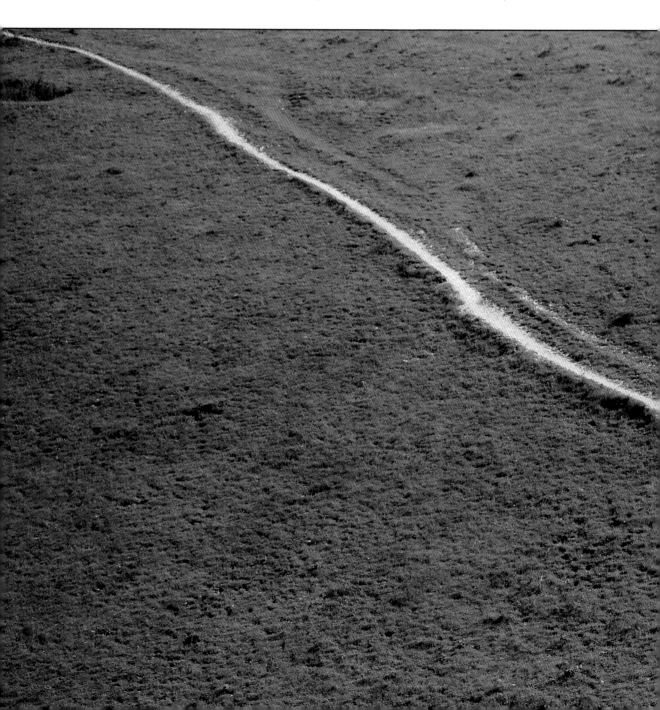

But when we put ourselves under the pressure of going for glory or striving for a personal best (PB), what physiological behaviour can we expect of our bodies? With our newly acquired physical and mental skills, how can we mitigate the stresses and strains when we make the leap into hard training sessions or racing?

Knowledge is, indeed, power, which is why I've always found it helpful to understand the detail behind how the body experiences the conditions under which it is required to perform. Obviously, a big influence on the physiological adaptations that take place during training is the type of fuel that we use, i.e. the food and beverages that we consume. This is a subject so huge that it merits a chapter in its own right, so turn to Chapter 9, Eat to win, for information on nutrition and to find out why the expression 'you are what you eat' is never so true as when tested in the sporting arena.

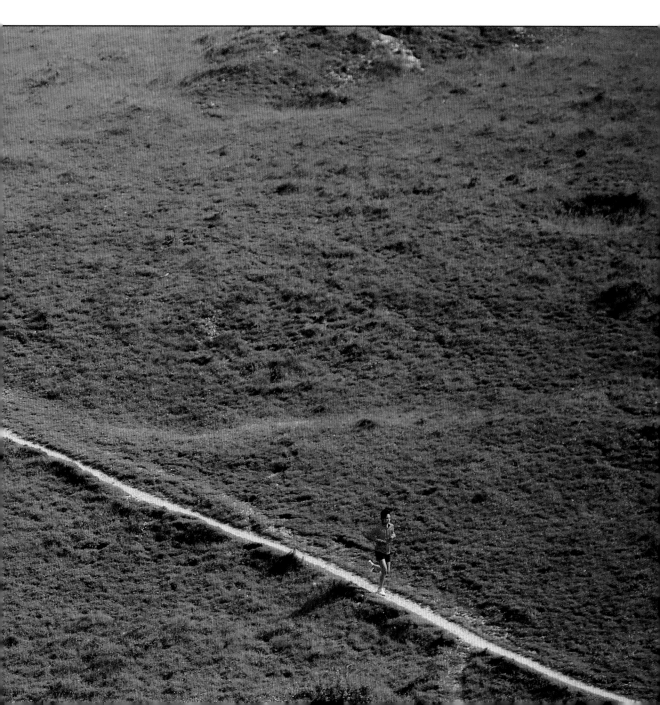

how the body adapts to training

As we gradually build up our mileage, what we're actually doing is training the body to become more efficient at running. We're also enabling it to make more efficient use of our energy stores in order to keep going for increasingly long periods of time.

WHAT VO2 MAX TELLS US ABOUT OUR POTENTIAL

One measure of our ability to do this is called 'VO2 Max', which you'll probably have come across in your reading or in conversation with fellow runners. Basically, it's a way of measuring how quickly and effectively your body can transfer the required energy to the muscles you're using, as and when you need it. The thinking goes like this:
• muscles need oxygen to perform;
• the more stress you place on your muscles, the more oxygen they need;
• therefore, the faster your body can exchange the waste carbon dioxide for oxygen and get it directly to your muscles, the better. So, a higher VO2 Max indicates a larger amount of oxygen consumed per breath and relayed to your muscles. In other words, the faster the muscles are provided with the oxygen they need (which they get from the blood circulation, a sort of oxygen 'larder'), the harder and better they'll be able to work and the faster you'll run. So it stands to reason that the higher your VO2 Max, the faster you'll be capable of running.

When we exercise, our muscle cells consume oxygen in order to be able to perform aerobic work. Using oxygen, the cells convert the energy we get from food into a different form of energy known as ATP. It's this that's used to power our muscles, and its production takes place in small 'power houses' within our cells, known as

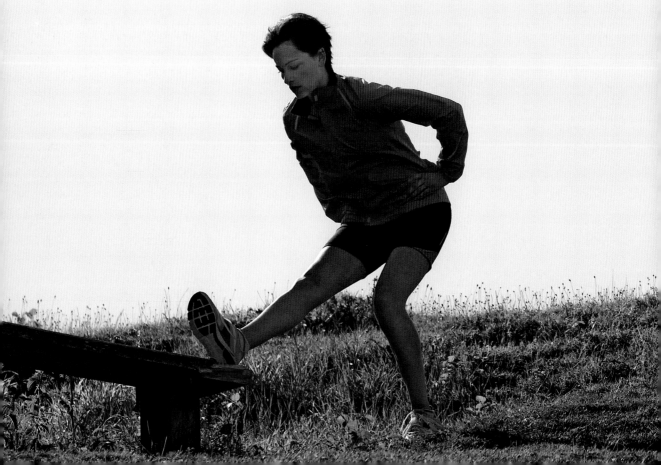

mitochondria. So, in order for muscles to work hard, they need an effective delivery system (the heart, lungs and blood circulation), as well as lots of mitochondria within the cells. One key effect of training is that we can increase the efficiency of our mitochondria in producing ATP.

THE DOWNSIDE OF VO2 MAX...

Although we can increase our VO2 max to some extent, genetics plays a huge role. Some people are born with a naturally high starting point for their VO2 – these people tend to make the best endurance athletes. On top of this, our genes determine the proportion by which we are able to increase our VO2 through training. For some people, training hard can lead to big gains; for others, less so.

THE HEART IS A MUSCLE, TOO

The muscle that we often don't think of as a muscle at all is the heart. In fact, it's the heart that responds best of all to training. It works the hardest during cardiovascular exercise, pumping the blood that carries oxygen and other nutrients to our muscles so that they can perform at their best. This is why a well-conditioned runner's heart will be larger and pump a higher volume of blood per heartbeat, providing more oxygen to the exercising muscles; these, in turn, are then able to work even harder. It starts to happen in a surprisingly short space of time – you'll see some changes in as little as four to eight weeks of consistent training, although the best effects tend to happen over a period of six months or more.

If training makes your heart work more efficiently, then logically, there must be a spin-off effect on the blood circulation, veins and arteries. When you're at rest, around 20% of your blood flows to your muscles; but when you're training hard it goes up to about 80%. The arteries in the muscles expand to allow more blood to flow through them, which carries additional oxygen and nutrients to the working muscles. From there, the blood gets pushed into the tiniest blood vessels known as 'capillaries'. When you're not exercising, the flow that goes through them is only small; but as you get fitter and stronger with training, they increase in number by up to 40%, enabling even greater amounts of oxygen and nutrients to assist the muscles with their task, as well as speeding the removal of waste build-up, such as lactic acid.

When you consider this process, you'll understand the importance of the cool-down (note: sometimes you'll hear it called 'warm-down'). If you've been training very hard and you suddenly stop, the heart's pumping action abruptly goes from flat out to very slow. This has a knock-on effect on your blood circulation, causing it to suddenly slow down, too. The net result is that there isn't enough pumping action going on to get the blood back to the heart and lungs again. The lungs are ultimately how we clear the lactic acid out of our systems, so if you continue to move around gently after you have finished exercising, rather than stopping still, you're actually assisting this process. What's more, stopping suddenly causes blood to pool in the leg muscles, which can make you feel light-headed, as though you're about to faint. Jogging slowly until your heart rate gradually slows to near normal is the best way to do this. A cool-down is a must!

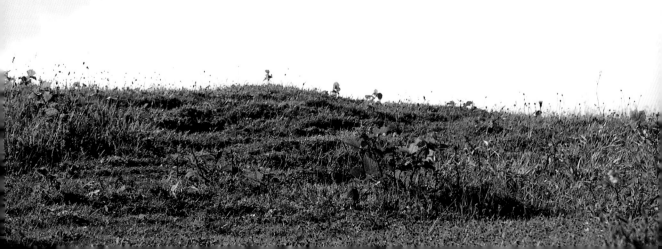

look after your immune system

The immune system is a complex mix of all sorts of different types of cells that go by tongue-twister names such as lymphocytes, leukocytes, immunoglobulins, eosinophils and, the most menacing-sounding of all of them, natural killer cells.

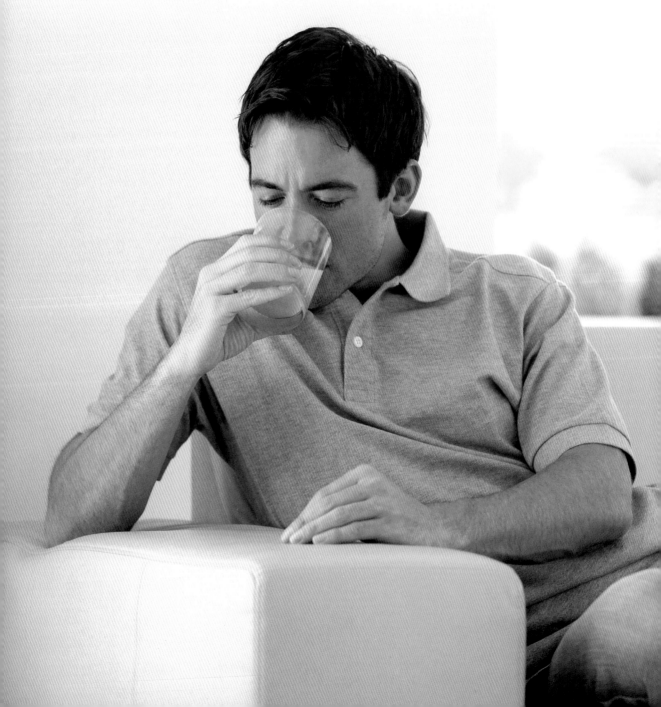

Many of these have their own specialised function, performing vital search-and-destroy missions to overwhelm foreign bacteria and kill parasites, tumours and viruses.

In the early 1990s, a research team led by Dr J Duncan MacDougall at McMaster University, Ontario, studied the effects on runners' immune systems of a variety of progressively tougher training programmes. Their results were published in August 1995 in *Medicine and Science in Sports and Exercise*. They found that runners' immune systems were depressed by an increase in the intensity of their training and that this was most noticeable at the start of a tough phase. As their training progressed, however, and their bodies adapted to the greater load and physical stress levels, their immune system adapted, too: they found that it returned to normal within 24 hours (although it can take up to 72 hours after a particularly hard-run event).

Obviously, no two immune systems are identical, so what brings down one runner may make no difference to another. Clearly, however, we're most likely to be at risk of succumbing to infection and illness in the early stages of increased intensity of training. So it's easy to see that we put ourselves at greatest risk if we over-train or increase our training too rapidly. Yet another good reason for building up gradually and allowing the necessary physiological adaptations to take place, rather than shocking our systems with sudden overload.

GIVE YOUR IMMUNE SYSTEM A BOOST

The first two variables that have a major impact on the efficient functioning of your immune system are nutrition and rest. Nutrition is covered in depth in Chapter 9, Eat to win, so suffice it to state here that when you combine hard training with poor food choices, you're heading towards crash and burn. My mantra is always to refuel with fluids, carbohydrate and some protein within 20–30 minutes of finishing training. This is the window in which your body can take that fuel and use it for muscle glycogen and immune system support as efficiently and beneficially as possible. Beyond this obvious point, read on for a few other reminders…

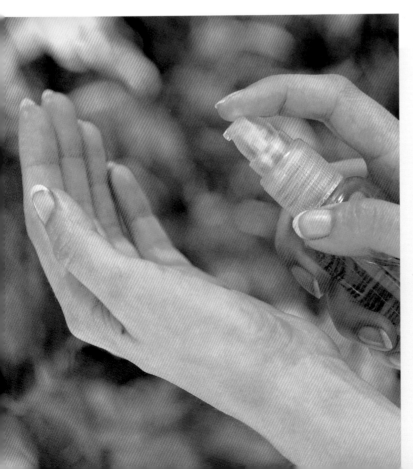

protect yourself

Get into the habit of limiting your daily exposure to bugs and viruses. During hard training your immune system is temporarily weakened, so it makes sense to avoid people with coughs and colds. Beware, too, the social practice of kissing friends hello and goodbye; even they don't know if they're harbouring a virus that has yet to make its presence felt. They know you, so they'll understand when you explain that you're gearing up for a forthcoming race.

You can also limit the physical access of bugs to your body by regularly washing your hands throughout the day or using an alcohol hand gel.

A big percentage of bugs are picked up on our hands from the surfaces we touch. This is why we should clean them when we've been working in an office or travelling on public transport – any environment in which we've been in contact with people.

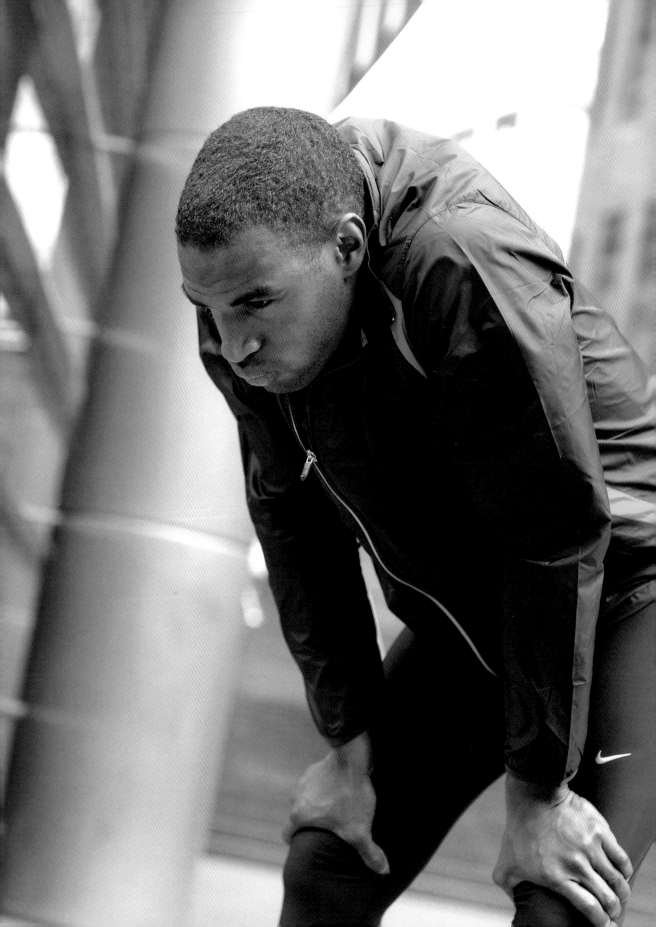

DON'T TRAIN WHEN YOU'RE UNWELL!

Picture your immune system frantically marshalling its resources to repel the invader (a virus) that's threatening to overwhelm it. What it's doing is mobilising the considerable energy that this process requires and throwing everything at the virus. Is it sensible, then, to ask your body to cope simultaneously with the stress of training or running a race, when it's already stretched to its limit fighting off a virus? The answer is an emphatic no.

The commonly agreed view is that minor ailments such as a mild cold or sore throat require little more than a day off to allow recovery, followed by some easy training and a watchful eye on how it goes. Anything more than this, such as aches, fever, headaches or extreme fatigue, steer clear of exercise altogether, stay away from other people (who won't thank you for passing any bug on to them), switch off your phone and put yourself to bed.

However, this does leave the definition of the common cold open to question. The obvious symptom is a runny nose, and continuing to train with just this on its own is fine; but if it comes accompanied by headaches and a generally achy, run-down feeling, then stop training completely. Or, to put it another way: if there's anything wrong above the neck, proceed with caution; below the neck and systemically (i.e. a feeling of general unwellness throughout the whole body), don't risk it – rest until you're better. Your body needs time to recuperate and repair itself. Everybody is different, so this could take up to a week or it could take longer. Once the illness has run its course, you can slowly get back to training. Be strict with yourself and do very little in the first week back, and only a little more than that in the second week. If everything goes according to plan, you're feeling great and sleeping well, then you can usually resume normal training in week three.

One thing we know for certain: if you try to train through it, or come back to exercise too quickly and with too much effort straight afterwards, you can push your body and immune system to breaking point. At best, you'll have a relapse or become more ill; at worst, you risk suppressing your immune system and putting yourself out of action for considerably longer – possibly even for years. Training while you're fighting a serious virus can bring on post-viral fatigue syndrome, also known as chronic fatigue syndrome or myalgic encephalomyelitis (ME). Many of us

know someone who has suffered from this depressing condition and watched their struggle with its debilitating symptoms: muscle and joint pain, a severe 'flu-like feeling, desperate tiredness, chronic sore throat, and poor memory and sleep patterns. For the sake of a few days off, it's really not worth the risk.

DEAL WITH THE RESOLVABLE ISSUES AND DITCH THE REST

Most of us don't have the luxury of being able to train full-time. We have jobs to go to, family to provide and care for, plus a host of responsibilities against which we either deliver or suffer the consequences of not doing so.

Inevitably, we sometimes have to deal with emotional matters that don't seem fixable. Make no mistake: once we open the door and allow these problems in, we risk having our minds colonised at a time when we're training hard and need a cool head and the space to switch off. Detachment from worry is widely acknowledged as necessary for the immune system to flourish and protect our health. Although a little bit of stress can actually make us more alert and act more quickly and more efficiently in the short term, too much of it is most definitely a drain. We all know that when we are stress-free we feel and look healthier.

There is only one way to cope with energy-sapping issues: deal with them. Where resolution isn't immediately possible, unpack the problems and take a long, hard, rational look at them. Identify and action any aspects that a) can be resolved right now; b) can be steadily worked away at; and c) cannot be dealt with immediately. Then pack c) away and get on with those of life's challenges that are achievable. Impossible? Not once you just get down to sorting things out. It takes resolve and determination, yes, and daily self-reminders (not dissimilar to the self-talk we looked at in Chapter 7, Mind games) each time problems threaten to invade our headspace, but it is do-able.

Mental techniques of this sort plus, of course, just heading for the great outdoors and getting on with running will help clear our minds, sharpen our perceptions and enable us to see life from a fresh perspective. The outcome that we're looking for is acceptance of the unalterable fact that we can only do what it is possible to do; and recognition of the futility and energy waste of stressing about things that are beyond our control.

feeling the burn

I've touched on lactic acid in previous chapters, but it's worth mentioning again in the context of how the body behaves in training and competition. A by-product of hard training, it's a sign that your body is working to keep up the momentum. Learn to handle lactic acid and you'll see the benefits.

There's a lot of confusion on this subject. It's often seen as the athlete's No.1 enemy, striking when there isn't enough oxygen available to the working muscles, and responsible for cramps and muscular exhaustion. It's a bit complicated, but if you want to know how it works, read on…

The energy we need for powering our muscle cells is provided by the breakdown of a molecule called adenosine triphosphate (ATP). The body has very limited stores of ATP, so we need to keep reassembling it so that it can carry on providing our energy. When we're running, we usually do this using oxygen (aerobic exercise).

The body uses glucose as its primary fuel source, but when there's no oxygen around (anaerobic exercise, e.g. sprinting), hydrogen ions build up. These ions are acidic – they are usually mopped up by another molecule called nicotinamide adenine dinucleotide (NAD), but when there isn't enough oxygen, NAD can't clear away the acidic ions, which explains the burning sensation in our muscles.

Fortunately, there's yet another molecule called pyruvic acid that can step in and move the offending ions away from the muscles into the blood stream in the form of lactic acid. When the lactic acid eventually lets go of the acidic ions, what's left behind is lactate: this can then be used as a further fuel source. The body clears the ions once there's enough oxygen again. If you've ever come across the term 'the oxygen debt' in your reading, this is what it means!

work with it, not against it

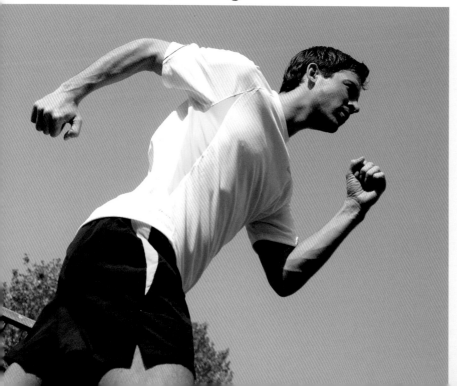

lactic acid facts

- Initially, the body gets its energy supplies from carbohydrate – this starts off the production of lactic acid. If needed, this can later be converted into glucose to be used when required.
- As a race gets tougher, the body uses its lactate supply as a fast-acting fuel source.
- The heart, slow-twitch muscle fibres and the diaphragm actually prefer lactate as fuel.
- In endurance events, the sensation that is called 'getting your second wind' refers to the effect of lactate kicking in.

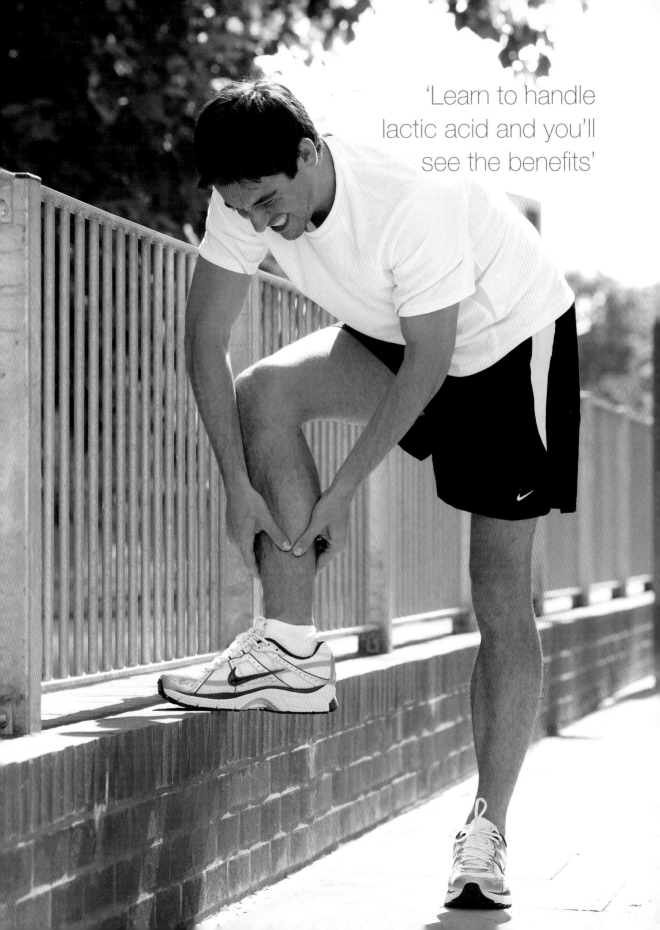

'Learn to handle
lactic acid and you'll
see the benefits'

dealing with muscle cramps

Some of you may already be familiar with this nightmare scenario: you're running along feeling quite comfortable, when wham, you get pulled up short by a painful knotting sensation. Sometimes it's more like a progressive tightening of a muscle that gradually slows you down.

This happens when a muscle contracts on its own, without your command. There are various types and causes, starting with the common-or-garden side stitch, which we've all experienced at one time or another. This is often caused by fast, shallow or irregular breathing and can usually be eased with deep, regular breathing. Then there's cramp caused by poor food and hydration management – depleted magnesium, sodium or potassium levels, for example. Then there's also the warning shot across the bows when cramp signals muscle damage. If you suspect it's the latter, do not continue running – seek medical help immediately. Let's look at some of these in a bit more detail.

Dehydration: Maintaining the correct balance of electrolytes (chiefly sodium and potassium, but also magnesium) and water is crucial to enabling our cells and organs to function. One such function is the regulation of the amount of water in the body. When you haven't drunk enough you'll have too high a concentration of electrolytes in the muscles, which can bring on cramp. If you start to feel any of the symptoms of dehydration, get out of the sun and top up your fluids. (Read more in Chapter 9, Eat to win.)

Over-hydration: On the other hand, if you drink too much water you can flood the cells and organs and tip the balance of electrolytes too far the other way by diluting your body's supply of salts, ending up with an insufficiency. This condition is called hyponatremia.

The key, always, is balance. Work out the hydration levels that are right for you in training so that you know how your body behaves and nothing is left to chance on race day.

Food intake: You'll have tried and tested food types and quantities to find out what works for you, but do remember that you shouldn't eat too close to the start of any major physical effort. Firstly, you don't want your blood supply diverted from your muscles to assist your digestive system just when you want all hands on deck to power your effort. Secondly, apart from the possibility of stomach cramp, you could also waste valuable time throwing up! Everyone will have worked out their own rules here, but generally, eat a small meal no later than three hours before your event or training session. Top up, if you want, with an energy bar or snack within the hour before you run, but only if you've tried it in practice with no problems.

pre- and post-run ritual

As I said in Chapter 3, Taking care of your body, a warm-up and stretch before the start is absolutely essential, especially if you anticipate a hard run in pursuit of a PB, or to gain a place among the front-runners. This is even more important after you've finished in the form of your cool-down and stretch. Although there's a cost involved, a sports massage is an excellent way to loosen up the muscles after a hard event or training session/week.

Too much effort, too quickly: If you expect your body to deliver Formula 1-type acceleration without having put in the training, you can also expect your muscles to protest. They are very likely to do this by cramping. Work up to your planned race pace in training before you give it a go in competition. *Always* warm up and cool down!

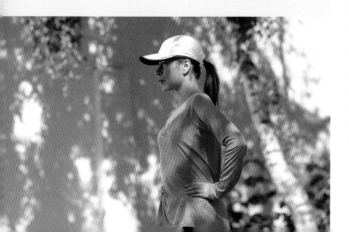

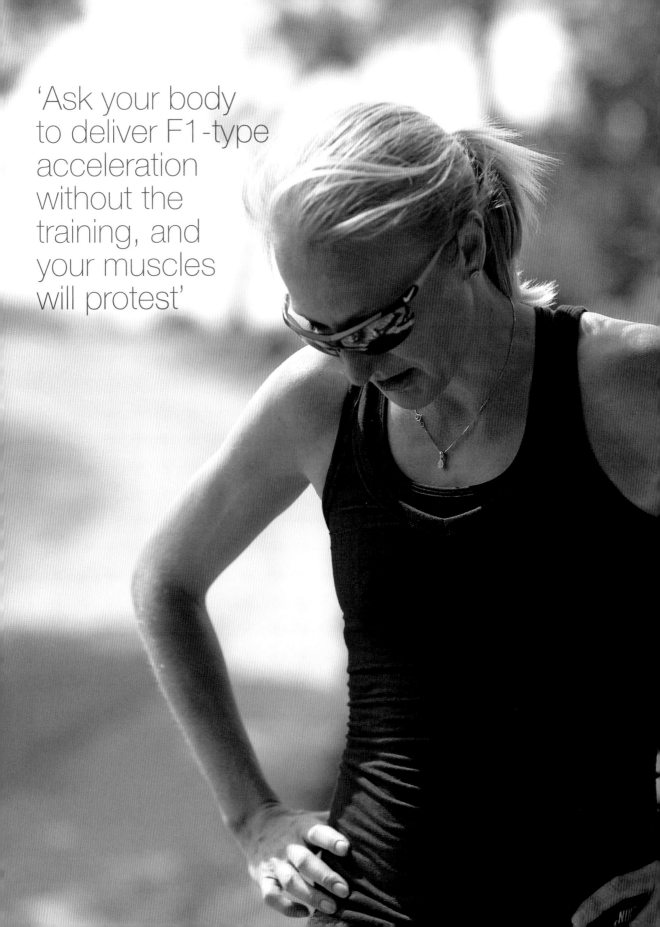

'Ask your body
to deliver F1-type
acceleration
without the
training, and
your muscles
will protest'

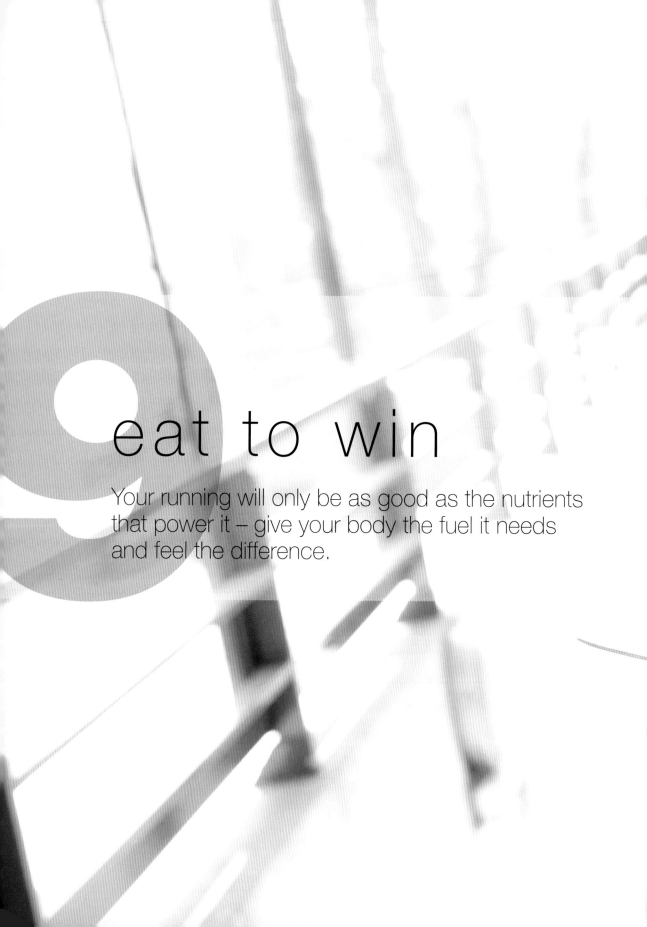

9 eat to win

Your running will only be as good as the nutrients that power it – give your body the fuel it needs and feel the difference.

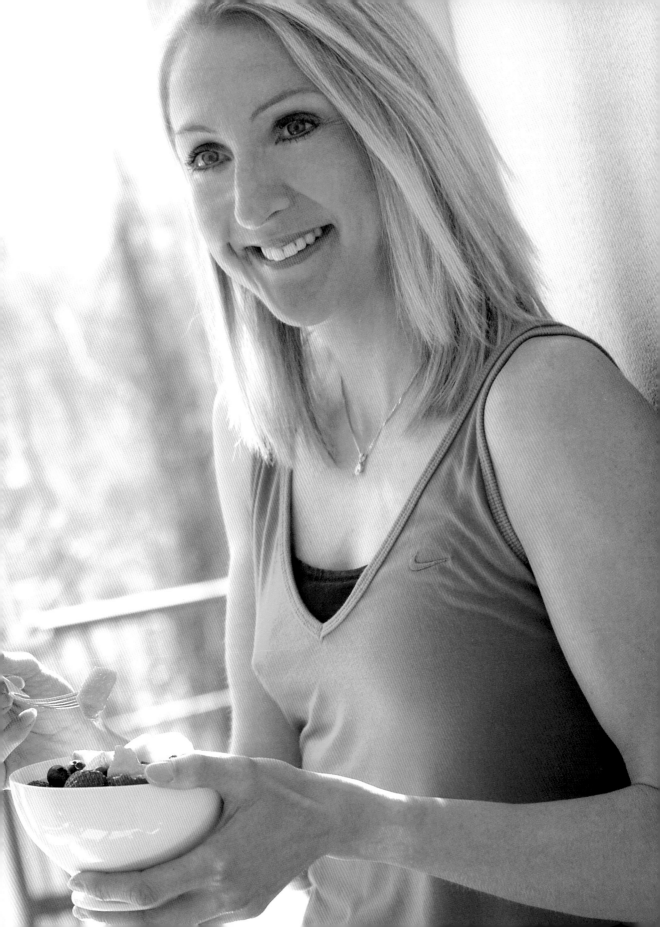

get your fuelling strategy right

If Napoleon did, indeed, say 'an army marches on its stomach', he was ahead of his time. No wonder the French did so well for so long. Eventually, their enemies started destroying food resources as they retreated – famished, the French soon lost their appetite for warmongering.

It's a good illustration. Our brain, nervous system, organs, musculature and skeleton depend entirely on obtaining the nutrients we need in order to heal and repair the body – in fact, to function at all.

If that's what's required in normal everyday circumstances, think how much more crucial it is for runners putting themselves through rigorous training regimes. I often hear people say that they're doing everything right in training, yet they're still struggling to get results. If you're among them, then one aspect that's worth taking a closer look at is your diet.

This chapter is all about how to fuel yourself properly, but let me set out my own stall before I begin: I'm a great believer in all things in moderation. We're humans, not machines. Life is for living, not for punishing ourselves – so if there's dark chocolate around, for example, you won't find me saying 'No thanks'.

What I've done here is try to group together the nutritional information that you might need to know for training purposes. I've set it out as a reference into which you can dip in and out as you need to. But I'm certainly not advocating a boot-camp approach to nutrition! With that in mind, read on.

KEEP A FIVE-DAY FOOD DIARY

There's only one way to keep a proper track of the nutrients you're putting into your body: write them down. Half of what we consume is what I call mindless nibbling – grazing while standing at the fridge, or snacking while chatting to friends in the pub. So, as an exercise, record the details of the food and beverages you consume over a five-day period. Include a weekend, as we all eat differently when we're not at work. Carry a notebook or use your mobile phone's note-taking facility. If you stop for a snack, make a note of it: tuna mayo sandwich? Okay, what type of bread? Salad, fine, but what was in it? Two cups of tea, great – with or without sugar and milk? What about the birthday cake that went round the office? How much non-caffeinated (and non-alcoholic) fluid did you have each day?

While you're at it, jot down the timings of your snacks and meals, with any relevant comments, especially in relation to before and after your training. This information could be useful should you need to look back and see whether there's a link between particular foods or not having eaten or drunk enough and any lethargy or other symptoms you may have felt a couple of days after a long run. Once you're fully aware of what you're consuming, you can make adjustments.

Looking at it later will give you an idea of how much protein, carbohydrates and fats (macronutrients) your diet includes. Within that, you'll be able to look at the proportion of fibre, vitamins and minerals (micronutrients). You'll also be keeping a record of how much fluid you drink. This will quickly tell you whether you're eating enough, what's missing and what's in excess.

Obviously, the quantity will depend on the level of intensity of your training. Advanced runners, whose programmes entail more speed work and longer weekly distances than people new to running, will fuel themselves accordingly. Essentially, you need to make sure you eat enough to replace what you use in exercise and to cover what you need for recovery. If your weight drops too low, your immune system won't function as effectively, plus you'll risk deficiencies of key nutrients that will get in the way of good performance. There are a number of websites you can use to calculate your personal calorie intake, such as the downloadable calculator you'll find on http://www.brianmac.co.uk/nutrit.htm

Also, as you'd expect, iPhone offers an array of clever apps for runners. Check out http://www.rncentral.com/nursing-library/careplans/50_iphone_apps_for_runners and be amazed. Warning: you'll be browsing for hours.

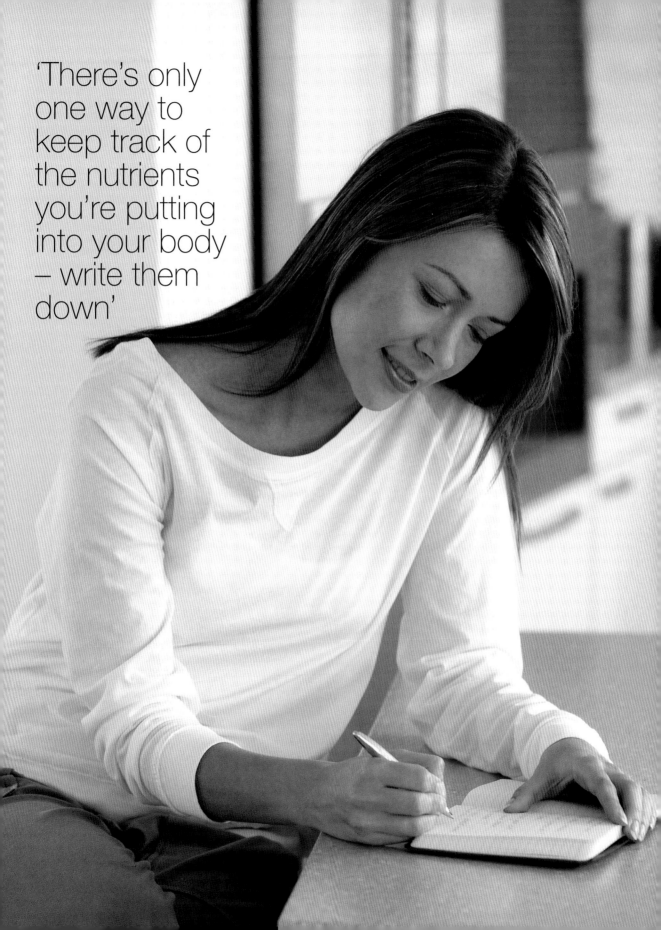

'There's only one way to keep track of the nutrients you're putting into your body – write them down'

when to eat

Remember your mother telling you to eat three square meals a day and not to snack in between? Forget that! The ideal is five smaller meals with three to four hours in between. Don't let this become an obsession, though – there are bound to be hectic days when it's impossible.

These days are no big deal. Carry a good-quality protein bar, or nuts, seeds or dried fruits, as a standby.

The main reason for eating less but more often is to keep your metabolism (the speed at which we burn up the fuel we eat) topped up and a continual supply of nutrients on tap to help with muscle repair. This also stops you getting so hungry that you over-eat when there's a chance.

BEFORE YOU TRAIN OR RACE

You can't run on empty, so it's crucial to make sure you get the macronutrients you need in good time before you exercise. If you're preparing for a long race, you need to build up your glycogen stores: start increasing your carbohydrate intake in the three days leading up to the race from 50–60% of your diet to between 70–85%. Also, research has shown that carbohydrates convert to glycogen (the fuel that powers your performance) more effectively when accompanied by water. No need to go overboard on huge carbohydrate-based meals – you'll just arrive at the start feeling bloated. Rather, pad out your main meals with extra carbohydrate and add in carbohydrate-based snacks.

On race day, this means a light but calorie-dense, carbohydrate-based meal three hours beforehand, with a smaller snack or energy bar/drink an hour before you run in order to top up your glycogen levels. You need to allow food time to be processed before you run. Using insulin as an example: its job is to clear carbohydrates out of the bloodstream and store them in the liver and muscles. But if you exercise too soon after eating, the insulin will still be hard at work clearing and storing, diverting the energy you need to power your performance.

AFTER YOU'VE TRAINED/RACED

Pay as much attention to replacing lost fluid, carbohydrate and protein as you did to fuelling up beforehand. Do this, ideally, within 15–30 minutes after completing your training session or race. Here's some technical information to shed light on what happens to your food when you

exercise. When you train hard, your muscles use…

- **glucose:** this is blood sugar that the body makes from the food you eat to provide you with energy;
- **glycogen:** any glucose you don't need for an immediate energy hit gets stored in the liver and muscles. This supply is called 'glycogen'. As soon as your glycogen store receives the signal that you've used up the glucose from your pre-race food intake, it releases some into the bloodstream to top up your energy levels.

If you've just completed a long and/or intense run or training session, your energy supplies will have plummeted and your muscles will have sustained some damage. This is a normal response to big physical effort. We know from research that the best time to kick-start the recovery process is within half an hour of finishing exercising. It's not always the time for a solid meal, though (and if you've just run your heart out, I doubt that you'll feel like it): choose a more easily digestible rehydrating liquid drink that contains carbohydrate and protein. Carbohydrate replaces your depleted glycogen, while protein helps with muscle repair and calms down the stress hormone, cortisol. If possible, include an easy snack such as an energy bar or banana, then try and get a good meal in the next two hours to optimise recovery.

You're not alone if you're thoroughly confused by the choice of protein drinks, bars and energy shakes. Everyone wants to know how to identify the good ones, but sadly there isn't one easy answer. Again, you'll have to experiment to find what suits you. Do try one of the natural sports bars before you try anything else. These are based on 100% natural ingredients and are free from additives, preservatives and artificial sweeteners. Look out for a minimum of 10g protein (ideally over 15g) per bar. Put back on the shelf those that contain stimulants such as caffeine or energy-giving herbs such as guarana or ginseng: they may not agree with you and, if you take them late in the day, could disrupt your sleep patterns.

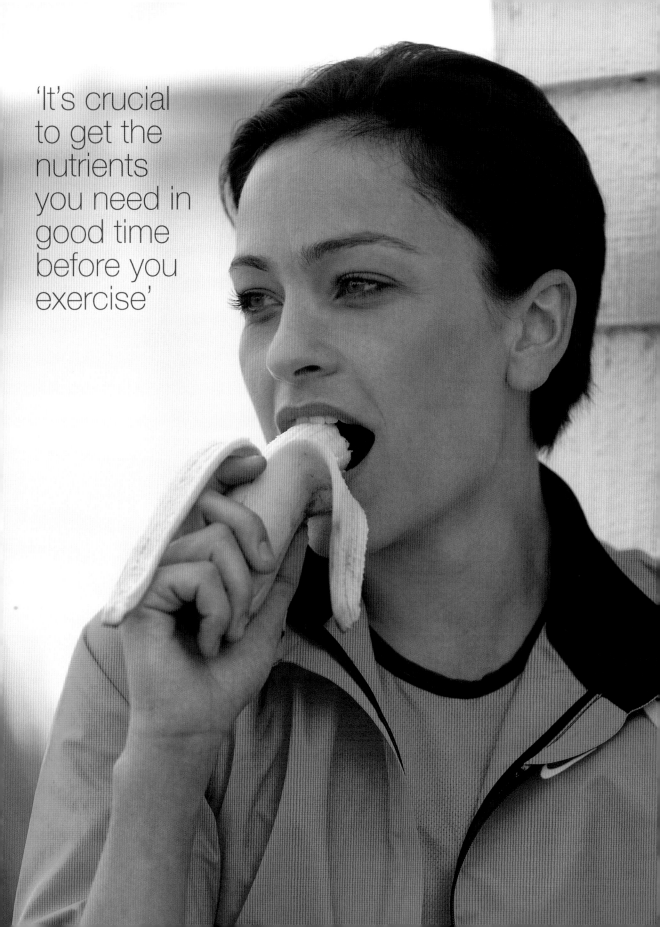

'It's crucial
to get the
nutrients
you need in
good time
before you
exercise'

what to eat

Okay, so we know when to eat to suit the demands of our training and racing schedules, but we also need to know what foods to choose to fuel the body and give us our best chance of success. Start by reviewing the ratio of carbohydrate/protein/fat in your diet.

CARBOHYDRATE

Most nutritionists agree that carbohydrate should form roughly half your diet. Bear in mind that food and beverage consumption varies greatly according to your size and the amount of training you're doing, so these figures are purely illustrative. Admittedly, this bit of the book isn't the most entertaining, but I think it's useful to have this information as a reference:

- assuming an average daily intake of 2,500 calories (kcals), roughly 1,250kcals (50%) will be carbohydrate;
- 1g of carbohydrate = 3.75kcals, therefore…
- 1,250kcals = 333g carbohydrate per day

We're not talking about any old carbohydrate – after all, junk food is carbohydrate, but it's of such poor quality that it will do little to enhance your prospects of a good performance.

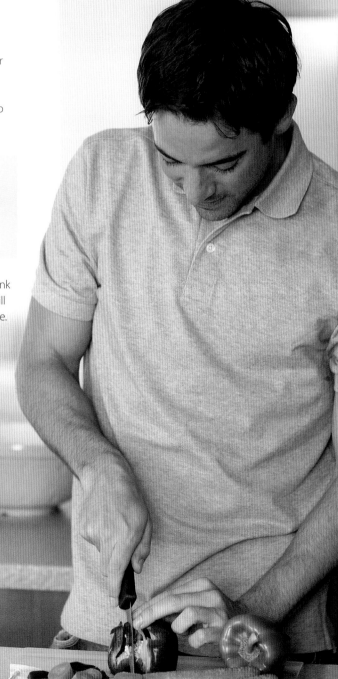

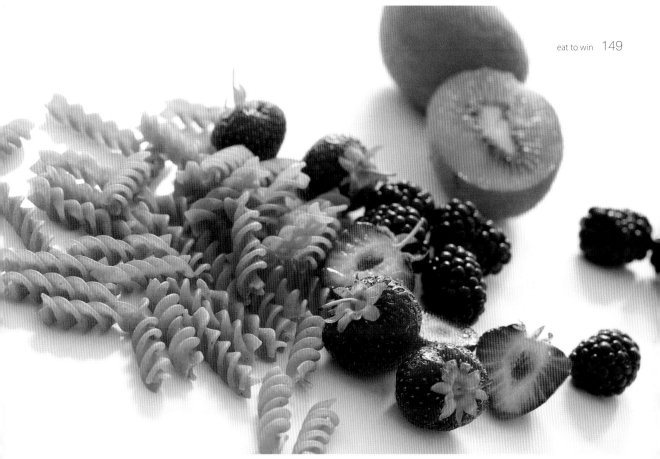

sources of carbohydrate

complex carbohydrates

These are the most important of the two, derived from fruit, vegetables and grains. The nutritional value of fruit and vegetables has been drummed into us since our first days at school, so no need to say any more here.

There is, however, more to say about grains. Choose unrefined, complex carbohydrates such as wholewheat breads and pasta, oatmeal, quinoa (pronounced 'keen-wa' – treat it like rice, it's delicious), bulgar wheat, buckwheat, barley, millet and brown rice.

Along with junk food, try to give a wide berth to highly refined food products. A good rule of thumb to keep at the front of your mind is that anything made from white flour (e.g. cakes, biscuits, white bread, white pasta, pizza and most proprietary breakfast cereals) lacks nutritional value. White rice also fits this category; it has had much of its natural goodness, fibre, vitamins and mineral content stripped out during the manufacturing process. The exception is basmati, which is ideal for loading before races and also for quick recovery, since it provides the fuel without the gastro risks that accompany high-fibre grains.

simple carbohydrates

Once again, it's refined foods containing sugar ('simple' carbohydrates) that are the baddies. Good sugar is found in fruit, for example, plus some vegetables and milk, whereas bad sugar (the sort sold in packets in shops), technically known as 'sucrose', is added to cakes, confectionery, biscuits, ice cream, desserts, fizzy drinks and a whole lot of ready-made products such as sauces. Sucrose causes sugar 'spikes' in your bloodstream, which upset the natural blood sugar balance and prompt a huge insulin response as your body tries to deal with it. The result is a brief rush of energy that quickly subsides, sapping your energy and leaving you flat and tired. However, let's not go overboard. After a hard run, a bit of sugar in moderation to help the body recover and reward your taste buds is not a bad thing. As a big fan of dark chocolate (well, it does contain good levels of magnesium and iron, as well as antioxidants!), I find that a few squares before training or before races does no harm at all, and neither does honey on my porridge.

If you've a sweet tooth and know you need to cut down, substitute a slightly more nutritious natural sweetener such as agave syrup or Sweet Freedom (made from apples, grapes and carob). These are sweeter than sugar, so you need less; they also have fewer calories and contain no artificial colourings, flavourings or preservatives.

PROTEIN

All the cell growth, repairs and building work that are continually being carried out in the body take place thanks to protein. Muscles, bones, hair, nails and skin – in fact, every single cell – contain it. Without protein we'd break down and stop functioning.

Very briefly, just so you have the facts: protein consists of 20 amino acids. The body manufactures 12 of them ('non-essential'), but there are another eight ('essential') that we can't make ourselves and have to get from food. But unlike carbohydrate and fat, we can't store protein in big enough quantities, hence we have to rely on our diet to provide it.

Exactly how much protein we need is a moot point; in any case, it varies between individuals. The elderly need more than younger people; athletes need more than sedentary folk; and body-builders need more than distance runners. Government guidelines recommend that men consume 44–55g of protein a day and women 36–45g. Nutritionists' guidelines recommend at least 1g per kg of bodyweight, and 1.2g–1.4g for moderate-to-heavy endurance training.

Studies have been done to work out how much protein is used up in distance running, usually by measuring the body's nitrogen balance (the amino acids in protein are the main source of nitrogen). In tests, runners' sweat, urine and faeces were tested for nitrogen loss at the end of periods of low-protein consumption, and again after periods of high-protein consumption. Results showed that runners need to consume more protein to maintain their nitrogen balance. This makes sense given how much extra repair work to muscles and capillaries is required after training or racing long distances.

There is loose agreement that protein should make up around 15% of your daily calorie intake. As I said, food and beverage consumption varies depending on your size and the amount of training you're doing; runners putting in huge training efforts will consume more, so this calculation is purely an example:

- assuming an average daily intake of 2,500kcals, roughly 375kcals would be protein;
- 1g of protein = 4kcals, therefore…
- 375kcals = 94g protein per day

THE HOLY TRINITY

Iron, zinc and magnesium are also essential for distance runners. The best source is high-quality lean, red meat; but if you're vegetarian, you'll need protein sources that also provide good levels of essential minerals – and you'll be eating around double what a meat eater would consume in order to make up your requirements. Examples of good sources of some or all three of these minerals are: avocado, blackberries, raspberries, dates, raisins, cherries, grapes, brussels sprouts, runner beans, potatoes, peas, pumpkin, asparagus, Swiss chard, nuts (especially cashews, almonds, Brazils, pine nuts and peanuts), oats, pumpkin and sunflower seeds, yoghurt and wheat, among others.

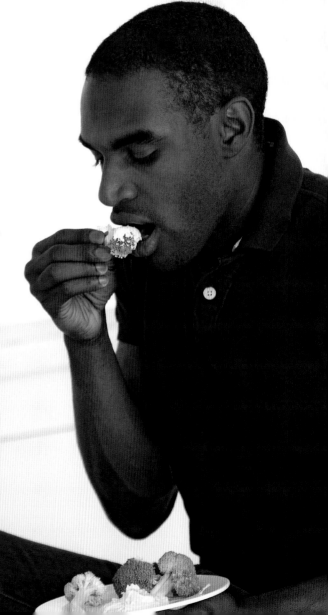

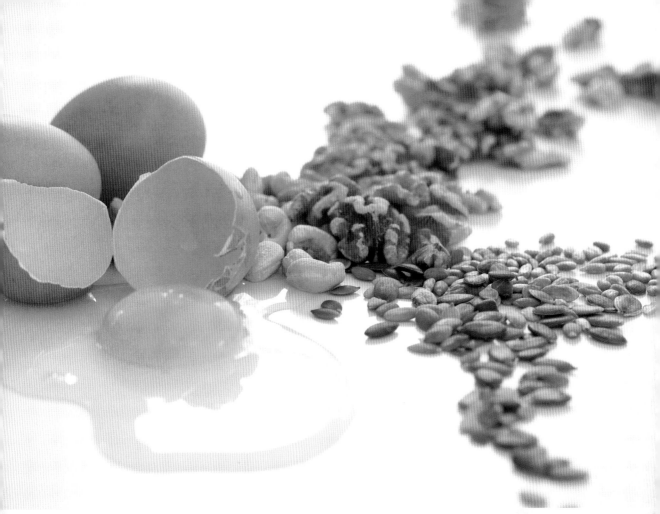

sources of protein

animal proteins

Animal proteins, as you'd expect, come from meat, poultry, fish, eggs and dairy – these contain all eight essential amino acids. A word of warning, though: some sources of high protein are also high in the wrong kind of fat (see 'Sources of fat' overleaf), so choose leaner cuts of meat or trim off visible fat. Roast, grill, steam or casserole to retain as much goodness as possible, and avoid deep-frying if you can. Having said that, dry frying (using a non-stick pan without oil) is good, and stir-frying with a high-quality olive or omega-rich oil such as flaxseed oil can help add good fats to your diet.

plant proteins

Plant proteins are found in:
- **Legumes and other vegetables**
  Peas, chickpeas, dried beans and baked beans, kidney beans, pinto beans, lentils, soya (including Quorn products), spinach, broccoli.
- **Nuts and seeds**
  Peanuts, walnuts, cashews, pumpkin, sesame and sunflower seeds, among others.
- **Grains**
  Rice, pasta, breads and anything else made from flour.

Between them all, these have plenty of amino acids, but none contains all eight to give you a complete protein source. This is why vegetarians and vegans need to plan their daily food intake to make sure they get the full quota. This is easily done by combining items from the grains category with something from either of the other three. Combinations might be baked beans/eggs with whole-wheat bread; humus with rice cakes/wholewheat bread; rice with lentils; wholewheat spaghetti with soya mince bolognaise; porridge with almonds and soya milk.

FAT

As a subject of conversation, fat is right up there alongside the weather, politics and footie. There's good reason. All fats are not created equal. Some are good for us (unsaturated fats); others are bad (saturated fats). Besides, fat contains almost double the number of calories as proteins and carbohydrates, so regardless of the health consequences, you can end up paying for your excesses by dragging around extra weight.

This is not to say that we can manage without fat altogether. We can't. It's the body's main energy source for low-intensity everyday activities such as sitting, sleeping, walking and desk work (high-intensity activity requires carbohydrate). What's more, without healthy fats, the body can't absorb and use vitamins A, D, E and K (which is why these are referred to as 'fat-soluble'). Fat also provides a protective barrier for our organs.

However, we don't require all that much of it; and we also need to distinguish between food sources that contain healthy unsaturated fats and those that contain harmful saturated fats.

The current view is that fat should be about 35% of our total food intake. Using the same illustration as before, this is what it looks like:

- assuming an average daily intake of 2,500kcals, roughly 875 kcals would be fat;
- 1g of fat = 9 kcals, therefore…
- 875kcals = 97g fat per day maximum (around 70g for women);
- of this, only 20–30g should be saturated fat (the lower figure applies to women and children)

A 2008 Food Standards Agency survey found that 80% of Great Britain is exceeding the recommended saturated fat allowance; the southeast shows an excess of 20%, with up to double the maximum allowance in the north of England and Scotland. This is not only contributing to the UK's obesity levels, it's also playing a part in the rise of coronary heart disease.

You may be thinking to yourself: 'But I'm a runner – I burn off everything I eat!' The reality is that even runners can still suffer the effects of excess saturated fat on their arteries, despite all the mileage and training they put in. Nutritionists report that they see a lot of people who believe they can simply counter the effects of what they eat by exercising, as opposed to adopting a healthy diet!

'All fats are not created equal. Some are good for us (unsaturated fats); others are bad (saturated fats)'

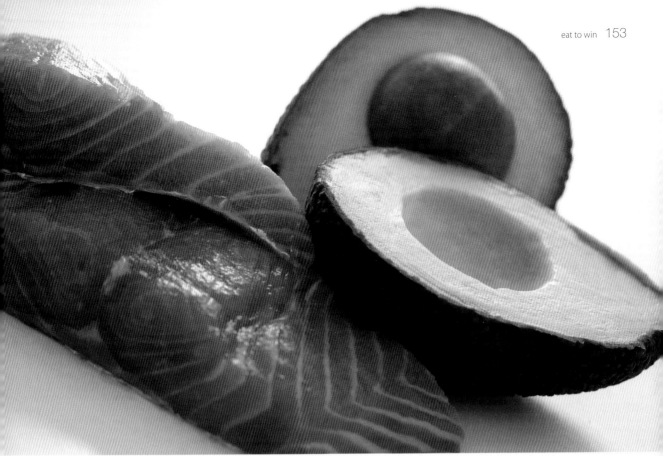

sources of fat

You can tell if fat is saturated if it's solid at room temperature: animal fats are the main unhealthy culprits here. Unsaturated, healthy plant-derived fats, however, remain liquid.

saturated fats

When I mentioned protein earlier in the chapter, I cautioned that some proteins are also high in the wrong type of fat. That's because saturated fat is found mainly in animal-derived foods. So, fatty cuts of red meat, sausages, fast foods (e.g. burgers, chips), poultry skin, cheese, butter, lard, cream, ice cream and full-fat yoghurt should all be consumed in moderation, i.e. less than 20–30g per day.

In this group, there is also one plant source of which we need to be aware: palm oil. It's high in saturated fat and it's used in a lot of manufactured foods. Another product that you may be surprised to hear is on the list is margarine: it's made from vegetable oil that is hydrogenised in manufac-turing. This process creates trans-fatty acids, a particularly harmful type of saturated fat that we should avoid totally. Yet transfats are everywhere – mass-market cakes, pastry and biscuits, crisps and fast foods frequently contain it. Trouble is, if you're reading this in the UK, at the time of going to press there is no requirement to show it separately on food labels. Get into the habit of reading labels before you buy, and keep an eye out for 'hydrogenated vegetable oil' – this often signals the presence of transfats.

unsaturated fats

Thankfully, this category of fats is beneficial, which explains the rave reports on the Mediterranean diet that we keep reading in the press. These come from fish and plant sources: avocados are full of it, as are nuts and seeds; fish rich in omega-3 such as salmon (wild is best), trout, sardines, mackerel and pilchards; oils (cold-pressed, if pos-sible) such as nut oil, virgin olive oil, sunflower and flaxseed oil.

In short, if you can replace your foods that contain saturated fat with foods containing unsaturated fats, you'll be doing yourself a big favour. Substitute one of the plant oils for butter and chuck out the margarine; eat more fish than meat; keep cakes and biscuits to a minimum; stick to grilling, steaming, dry-frying or stir-frying; and opt for low-fat dairy produce such as milk and yoghurt whenever possible.

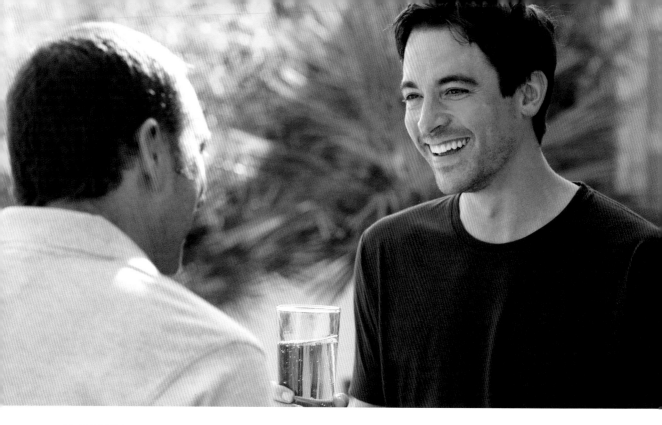

ALCOHOL

Although it gets its own section, it's the shortest one, because you know most of the facts about alcohol already!

By and large, alcoholic beverages have little, if any, nutritional value. However, the double whammy is that they are also high in calories. Stop off for a few drinks with friends on the way home and by the end of an entertaining evening you could find that you've used up half your daily calorie allowance! A pint of draft beer can contain anything from 140 kcals for a lager to 200 kcals for a stout. A glass of dry wine is around 106 kcals for a standard measure, but if it's dessert wine, make that a headache-inducing 226 kcals. Put away three glasses of wine over dinner and you've consumed an additional 300–400 kcals without even factoring in the food you've eaten. Spirits are just as bad: the higher the percentage proof (i.e. alcohol content) the more calorific it is. Standard mixes such as gin and tonic come in at 170 kcals, with a single shot of whisky around 70 kcals. Suddenly the term 'empty calories' has real meaning.

Remember, alcohol is a diuretic – it dehydrates you, which means it depletes your electrolytes. It also challenges your balance! The more training you do, the more finely tuned your body becomes, so even a couple of drinks can have this effect. Best to give large amounts of alcohol a miss if you're on the run-up to an event for which you've been training for ages. However, when all's said and done, a glass of red wine a couple of times a week is good for your heart and gives you some antioxidants, as well as being enjoyable; and if it helps you get a good night's sleep, so much the better. As I've said before, life is for living, so let's live a little!

FLUID INTAKE

This book is peppered with mentions of hydration because it's of such crucial importance to runners. Even when you're accustomed to keeping a watchful eye on your fluid intake you can come unstuck. This is usually due to logistics: you're out and about, you've forgotten your water bottle and it's not easy to get any.

As a general rule, we need at least 1.5 litres of fluid per day ('fluid' includes all non-alcoholic, non-caffeinated drinks). But that's just an average; the way to work out exactly how much you need for your size is to multiply your body weight in kilograms by .033. So, if we take someone weighing 56kg as an example: 56 x .033 = 1.8 litres. Plus, there's general agreement that runners need an extra litre for every hour that we run (more if it's hot).

In hot weather, pay attention to minerals in the fluid you drink and opt for rehydration rather than huge energy boosts. However, a specialist hypotonic drink will be a quicker, more effective way to rehydrate than plain water.

TO SUPPLEMENT OR NOT TO SUPPLEMENT?

The question everyone wants answered is: do I need supplements in addition to what I'm already eating? There are two schools of thought:

- If you know that you eat a healthy and balanced diet, you should be getting all the nutrients your body needs from your food.

As against:

- Modern farming practices have reduced the quality of our food to the point where we all need to supplement our day-to-day diets.

Which one is right? Well, there's no hard and fast answer, as it all depends on your individual circumstances. Do you know, for instance, whether you are deficient in any particular vitamins or minerals? Do you follow a selective diet such as veganism or vegetarianism? Do you have any allergies or intolerances, such as wheat, dairy or nuts? Are you anaemic?

It can be costly at best, and counter-productive at worst, to have a go at vague and sketchy self-diagnosis. However, if you do find that you are doing everything right –

i.e. you're not over-training or burning the candle at both ends, and you're eating adequately and healthily – yet you still feel constantly tired, fluey and take longer than usual to recover from training, then it's worth seeing the GP. A blood test will reveal any deficiencies that might be a factor.

However, it's worth remembering that the word 'supplement' means just that: a useful way to supplement a well-balanced diet, as opposed to a replacement for proper food. In theory, you get what you pay for: some brands are more expensive than others, but these are more likely to be composed of the most absorbable forms of nutrients with fewer binders and fillers.

As a general rule, runners need higher levels of vitamins and minerals to support their immune systems during training and racing. Unless you are one of the few whose diet is pretty close to perfect, I would suggest that you take a high-quality multivitamin and mineral supplement that contains good iron levels and an antioxidant complex. In order to ensure efficient calcium uptake from your diet, make a point of getting enough vitamin D: 20 minutes in the sun without sun cream with one fifth of your body exposed will do the trick. However, if you live in the UK, it's not a bad idea to consider a vitamin D supplement in the winter months.

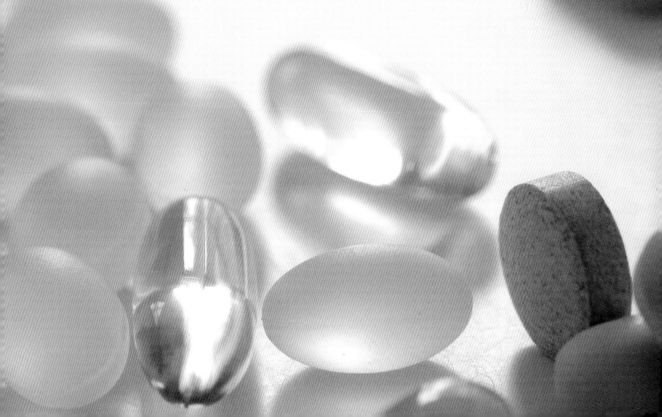

essential nutrients

If you take any medication, consult your GP before you start a supplement regime: there are contra-indications for some supplements when they are mixed with certain pharmaceutical drug treatments.

	what it does	where to get it
iron	Iron is key to making haemoglobin, which acts as the carrier of oxygen to the blood vessels and muscles; low levels will compromise performance and could lead to anaemia. A deficiency means fewer, much smaller red blood cells being produced than normal. However, true anaemia is quite rare: if you eat a healthy diet you probably won't experience it. The few runners who do are usually menstruating women and/or vegetarians, and those who are training at altitude. However, students leaving home for the first time and surviving on 'modified' diets can also be susceptible. If you feel that your symptoms are consistent with anaemia, go and see your GP who can determine it very quickly. Never attempt to self-diagnose – you won't know what form or dosage of iron supplement to take without a blood test, and it's not something about which you can hazard a guess.	There are two categories of source: heme (found in animal products) and non-heme (found in plant products). **heme**: lean red meat (especially liver), eggs, seafood (especially oysters, salmon and tuna), poultry to a lesser extent. **non-heme:** wheat, oats, lentils, soya, spinach, broccoli, dried fruit, blackstrap molasses (excellent energy-booster: 1 tablespoon of blackstrap molasses twice a day in warm water, milk, or on its own if you don't mind the taste).
vitamin C	This comes next on the list owing to its role in helping the body absorb the iron that's needed to carry oxygen to the muscles. It's an antioxidant that supports the immune system and assists with tissue growth and repair, as well as protecting against blood clotting and bruising; it also helps heal any damage from heavy training sessions.	Oranges, kiwi fruits, strawberries, tomatoes, broccoli, peppers, brussels sprouts, spinach.
vitamin E	Vitamin E, like vitamin C, is an important antioxidant, playing a major role in protecting the body's cells from damage caused by strenuous exercise, it also helps maintain a healthy heart, blood and circulatory system.	Avocado, asparagus, leafy vegetables (e.g. spinach), watercress, brussels sprouts; corn, olive, safflower and soya oils; nuts and seeds; wholemeal breads and wheatgerm; mackerel and salmon; blackberries and mangos.
the B vitamins	A good B complex supplement consists of B1 (thiamine); B2 (riboflavin); B3 (nicotinic acid); B6 (pyridoxine); B12 (cobalamin); and folic acid. This group helps with muscle repair and recovery, prevention of anaemia through supporting the production of red blood cells, as well as helping maintain energy levels and the immune system.	Yeast extracts (Marmite and brewer's yeast), meat, poultry and fish; broccoli, spinach, potatoes, avocado and bananas; dried apricots, dates and figs; milk, cheese, yoghurt and eggs; nuts and pulses; brown rice and whole grains.

what it does

where to get it

calcium

This is essential for muscle and nerve function, and also blood clotting. When you don't get enough calcium from your food, the body simply takes it from the next available source – your bones. This reduces their density, weakening them and increasing the risk of stress fractures. Under the age of 50, sedentary people need around 1,000mg per day; after that 1,200mg. Runners can afford to go higher: if you're exercising strenuously, you can take between 1,200–2,600mg per day.

However, I'd advise erring on the side of caution before you go bumping up your intake of vitamins and minerals beyond the recommended daily allowance. Too much can be as bad as too little, so see a nutritional therapist for a specialised supplement programme. And remember, calcium needs to be balanced with magnesium (about 1mg magnesium for every 2g of calcium) for optimum absorption.

Whole milk (a single glass contains 300mg; however, skimmed milk won't do it for you, and neither will soya milk unless it has 'Fortified with calcium' on the label); dark green vegetables (which also contain folic acid) such as spinach, broccoli, bok choi, asparagus, garlic; herbs like basil, dill, thyme, oregano, rosemary; tofu, quinoa and blackstrap molasses (there is greater calcium density in molasses than in dairy products).

magnesium

This is known as a 'major mineral', i.e. we need a daily minimum of 100g. It helps build strong bones, muscles and teeth and controls blood pressure. It's also crucial to the release of energy, because it's an essential component in the manufacture of ATP, the energy carrier in our cells that powers everything we do.

It has another role in helping absorb and break down other nutrients such as calcium and vitamin C. It's often taken with vitamin B6, as this increases the amount of magnesium that enters cells.

A sign of low magnesium can be persistently sore, aching muscles and easy bruising. However, it is possible to have too much of it: one of the side effects of large doses is diarrhoea, so seek advice before you start taking it as a supplement.

Green leafy vegetables (especially spinach), courgettes, parsnips, peas, sweetcorn, pumpkin and artichokes; figs, prunes and raisins; bananas and apricots; fish (tuna, pollock and haddock); meat and dairy produce; nuts (especially almonds, Brazils, cashews and pine nuts); buckwheat, quinoa, pearl barley, oats and brown rice; wheat bran (e.g. Weetabix, All Bran) and wheatgerm; pumpkin seeds, soya beans and tomato paste; dark chocolate!

omega-3

Known for its lowering effect on cholesterol, for runners it's the anti-inflammatory properties that will be of most interest.

Flaxseeds, walnuts, salmon, mackerel, scallops, tofu, tuna, cod, kidney beans, spinach, eggs.

zinc

You lose zinc when you sweat, so runners need to make sure they eat a diet rich in this metal. It is an important support for your immune system, as well as ensuring that the enzymes that regulate your metabolism and give you the energy you need are working efficiently.

Beef, pork, lamb, the dark meat of chicken, peanuts and peanut butter, fortified breakfast cereals, seafood (especially oysters), legumes.

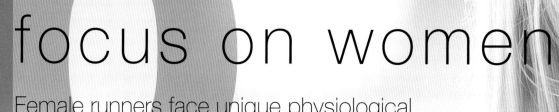

10 focus on women

Female runners face unique physiological
challenges. Get to grips with the practicalities of
dealing with them and you'll run with confidence.

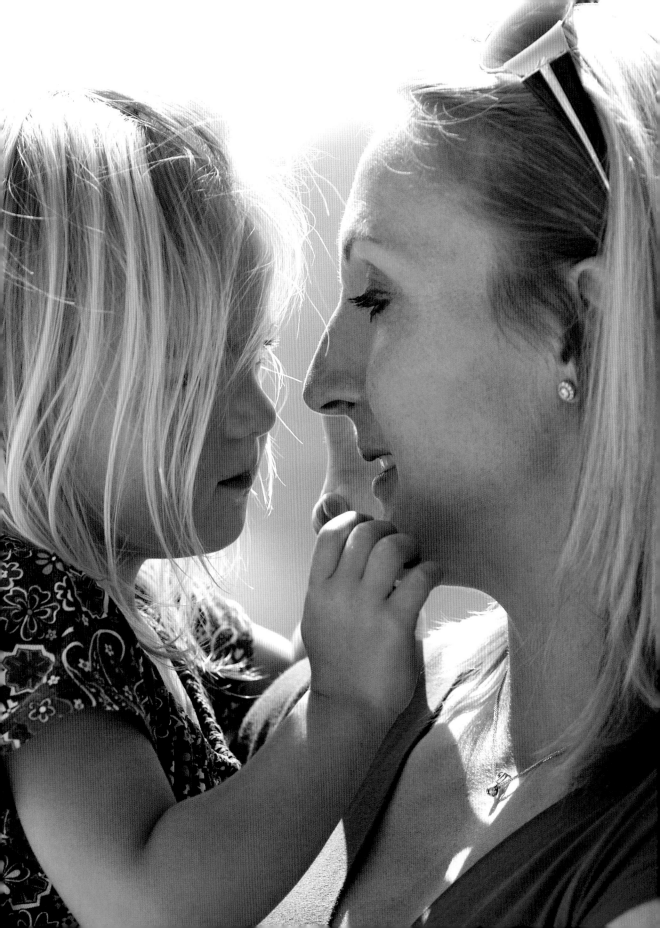

vive la différence

I was prompted to write a chapter focusing on women runners for some very practical reasons. Simply put, I believe that our physiological differences are such that separate consideration will boost our ability to perform at our best.

The journey from girlhood to womanhood offers pretty unique challenges for the young runner. For those who started running at a young age as I did, normal body changes can sometimes temporarily get in the way. For instance, the average normal weight gain for a maturing girl is 4.5–9kg; this is a prerequisite for regular menstrual patterns (nutritionists maintain that we need, on average, 17% body fat). Male athletes, meanwhile, can flourish on under 10%.

Structural differences include a wider pelvis (to facilitate childbirth). This, in turn, creates an inherent weakness in the anterior cruciate ligament of the knee, with which male athletes don't have to routinely contend. We have less muscle and haemoglobin, too, which means that male runners benefit from greater oxygen uptake. Plus, they have a more efficient heat dissipation system – they sweat more. We, on the other hand, 'radiate' through the skin, which means less blood moves through our muscles.

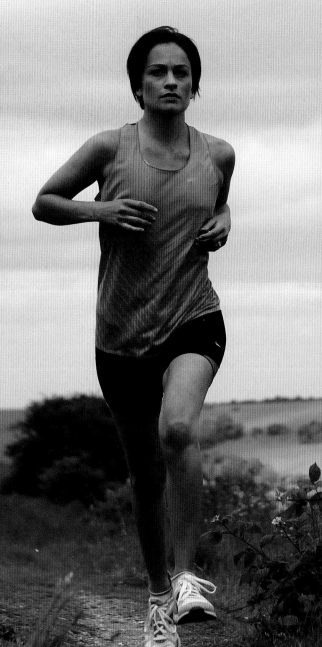

But at least all women experience these issues, which makes for a level playing field. That we can compete at all is thanks to a determined and talented few. We didn't participate in organised sport until the 20th century: the first international championship to schedule women's events was the 1928 Olympics. Having said that, the women's marathon didn't make it on to the roster until Los Angeles, 1984. It was won by Joan Benoit Samuelson in 2 hours, 24 minutes and 52 seconds, ahead of a class field that included Norway's Grete Waitz and Ingrid Kristiansen, and Portugal's Rosa Mota. But best of all, it finally put to rest the quaint notion that women were '… physiologically incapable of prolonged physical activity' (Lucas & Smith, 1982).

Of course, when brute strength and power are the only measures of success, clearly men, with their superior musculature, will come out on top. But research suggests that well-trained women can do equally well at ultra distances, when performance tends to even out (see Speechly et al, 1996). Does this herald an exciting future for women's distance running? Time will tell.

Meanwhile, let's look at the practicalities that confront women during their running careers and how best to deal with them.

'Research suggests that women can do equally well at ultra distances'

coping with 'The Curse'

Periods are sometimes thought of as a curse – indeed, it was often known as 'The Curse' by our mothers and grandmothers. Sure, it's an inconvenience just before a race for which you've trained your socks off; however, let's get it in perspective: it's a normal biological occurrence that affects all female runners.

Don't let it get in the way. Pack a tampon or two in your pocket and keep a couple in your kit bag for emergencies; if they suit you, tampons are the better bet because they're less likely to cause chafing. However, if you feel unsure and don't want the distraction of worrying, then wear a pad as well for extra confidence. As always, try this in training first.

There's no evidence to suggest that your performance need be handicapped by your menstrual cycle. On the contrary, there's a lot of anecdotal evidence to suggest that physical exercise actually helps alleviate cramps and water retention, thanks to the brain's release of the mood-enhancing chemicals, endorphins, plus better blood circulation. Not only do they make you feel mentally terrific, they have a handy pain-killing effect, too.

Personally, I feel worst in the few days before my period arrives: my legs are heavy and sluggish and I suffer from that bloated, water-retention feeling. To combat this, I conversely drink more water, avoid excess sugar and salt, take ice baths and get more rest. I actually set the first of my marathon world records in Chicago the day my period arrived. Once underway, I forgot all about it and, aside from a slightly unsettled tummy and some cramps after the race, I don't believe it got in the way at all. Anyway, I was determined not to let it affect my race after months of hard work.

COPING WITHOUT 'THE CURSE'

We can't look at menstruation without considering what happens when it stops. Although this does sometimes occur in sedentary women, there are rather more cases among athletes. Huge dedication often translates into extremely hard, high frequency training schedules; hence the greater likelihood of female athletes to be leaner than average. We also have a tendency to put ourselves under higher stress levels, which can temporarily halt ovulation.

Despite the fact that some nutritionists maintain that body fat needs to be 15–17% in order for menstruation to occur, I've maintained regular periods with body fat

of around 12–13%. There's a new school of thought that may shed light on why this is. It suggests that it's not your absolute amount of body fat that is important, but rather your calorie balance. If you're training hard on a calorie intake that's only just enough to meet your exercise requirements and no more, there's nothing left for the body to use to repair damage caused by the micro-trauma to the bones, muscles and soft tissues. This chronic state of very slightly under-supplying yourself with calories is not enough to make you lose weight, but it is enough to affect your hormonal balance. This has the effect of literally switching off your menstrual cycle, quickly leading to loss of bone mineral density, which can potentially result in fractures.

So, if you are naturally lean and train hard, but you eat enough to fuel your energy output and you get adequate sleep and rest, then your menstrual cycle is unlikely to be affected. But if you try to maintain a weight that's genetically too low for your body type by eating too few calories and generally short-changing yourself nutritionally, you'll become prone to amenorrhea.

There have only been two occasions in my life when my periods disappeared. The first was when I left home for university, but they would return like clockwork at term breaks; the second was after the Beijing Olympics. I believe that both instances were due to the increased stress at these junctures in my life. Our bodies are designed to survive, so under pressure they will prioritise energy output and conservation.

If you find that your menstrual cycle has become very erratic and/or stops altogether, ease back on your training; identify any increased stress in your life and reduce it; increase the quantity of (nutritious) foods that you eat; and see a doctor and/or nutritionist immediately. They may well recommend a bone scan now, with a repeat the following year, in line with current thinking on frequency for athletes.

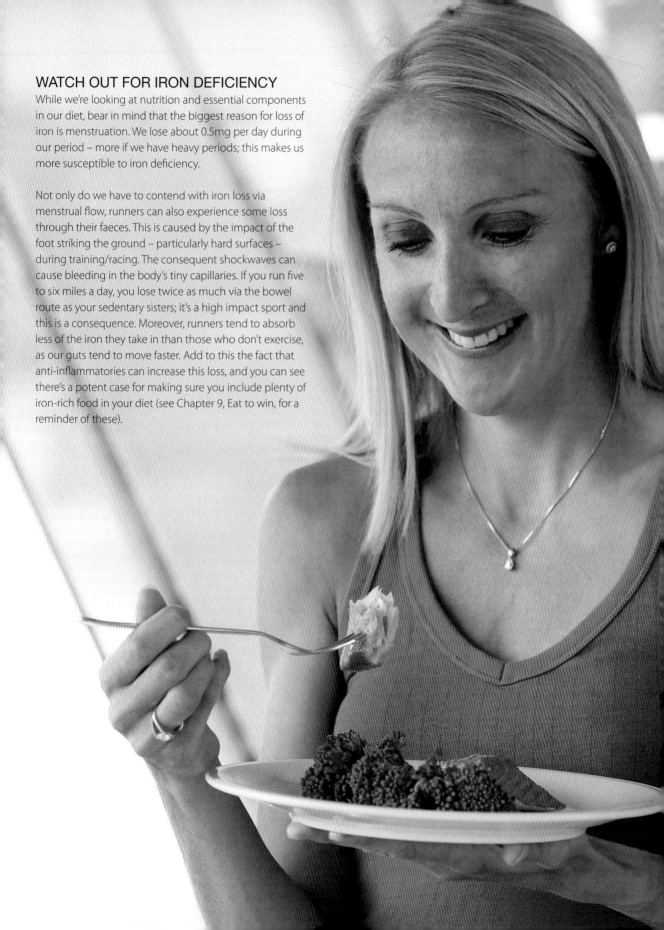

WATCH OUT FOR IRON DEFICIENCY

While we're looking at nutrition and essential components in our diet, bear in mind that the biggest reason for loss of iron is menstruation. We lose about 0.5mg per day during our period – more if we have heavy periods; this makes us more susceptible to iron deficiency.

Not only do we have to contend with iron loss via menstrual flow, runners can also experience some loss through their faeces. This is caused by the impact of the foot striking the ground – particularly hard surfaces – during training/racing. The consequent shockwaves can cause bleeding in the body's tiny capillaries. If you run five to six miles a day, you lose twice as much via the bowel route as your sedentary sisters; it's a high impact sport and this is a consequence. Moreover, runners tend to absorb less of the iron they take in than those who don't exercise, as our guts tend to move faster. Add to this the fact that anti-inflammatories can increase this loss, and you can see there's a potent case for making sure you include plenty of iron-rich food in your diet (see Chapter 9, Eat to win, for a reminder of these).

pregnancy and exercise

Looking back on how things were for our mothers and, certainly, our grandmothers, the very idea of exercising in pregnancy was considered eccentric and laughable at best, certifiable and dangerous at worst. Women 'with child' were fragile creatures who were encouraged to rest.

When I visited my gynaecologist five months into my first pregnancy, she somewhat freaked at the fact that I was running every day and occasionally twice a day! However, after the delivery she told me that from then on she'd be recommending exercise to all her mums-to-be. Today, we know all about the benefits of moderate exercise in pregnancy. Women feel healthier and stronger for it, while babies are more prepared for the stress of birth, have better muscle tone and are less likely to grow up overweight. It's also thought that they do better at school.

If you were running before (don't take up running when you find out you're pregnant!), then provided you're having a healthy, normal pregnancy and your doctor knows that you're still running, there's no reason to stop.

However, there are some crucial ground rules.
- if you experience any vaginal bleeding, abdominal pain or reduction in the movement of your baby, stop running immediately and seek urgent medical advice.

- If you have any pregnancy complications (e.g. raised blood pressure, protein in your urine or early signs of pre-eclampsia) again, stop running.

- Make sure you stay well hydrated; never overheat; keep your glycogen levels topped up; and, obviously, listen to your body. I can't emphasise this enough, especially in the first trimester when we feel so very tired. It's at this point that all the placenta and blood volume groundwork is being laid down, yet the foetus is so small that we often feel that it's an excuse, rather than a compelling reason, for taking it easy.

But if you're fit and healthy and you listen to your body, you will benefit from regular, manageable exercise. It will counter that insidious feeling of nausea, help you maintain a good weight and give you energy. Best of all, you'll have the enjoyment of your runs, plus you'll recover faster after your baby's arrival.

IT'S OKAY TO WORK OUT

In the first trimester, there's barely any discernible difference in your body shape, but fatigue, nausea and an increased blood volume (hence lower haemoglobin and red blood cell levels) sometimes make this a tough time. So, don't push yourself – your body has a lot to cope with, so rest is crucial. Throw time and route calculations out of the window: running now is totally different from how it is for the non-pregnant you, so no more diary comparisons!

Thankfully, the second trimester is often when you feel at your most active, but it's also when you need to slightly modify your exercises as your belly grows.

There's general agreement that around half an hour's daily exercise is optimal. I'm not talking about full-on training here – that should be modified, lessened in intensity and limited to four sessions a week. After four months, however, avoid exercises that involve lying flat on your back: it's linked to decreased cardiac output (i.e. a reduction in the volume of blood pumped by the heart due to pressure on the vena cava, the largest vein in the body). It goes without saying that this is neither good for you nor your baby. Similarly, your centre of gravity shifts as you gain extra weight during the course of your pregnancy, and ligament laxity begins in readiness for the stretch required for baby's exit. Women sometimes report a dull ache in the small of the back, sacro-iliac pain and, occasionally, stronger back pain. Strong abdominal and core muscles will go a long way to reducing this; but if you haven't built these up before your pregnancy, now is not the time to start. Indeed, excess abdominal exercises with a growing belly are not recommended! This can cause the left and right sides of your abdominal muscles to separate, leaving a gap between them, a process known as 'diastasis recti'. This muscle separation is not generally the result of tearing or rupture, rather they simply thin out, so there's little pain. But continuing to do tough abdominal exercises if your stomach muscles split can lead to the problem worsening and a reduced chance of them re-knitting post partum.

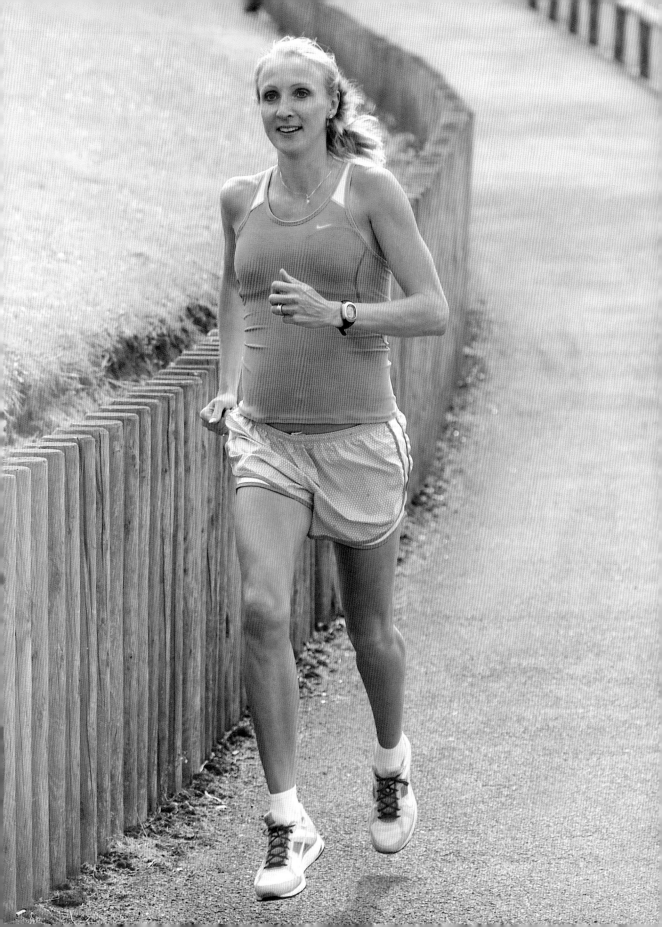

WHAT ABOUT WEIGHT-TRAINING?

If you were training regularly with weights before you were pregnant, there's no need to stop now. But once again, common sense must prevail: it's not the time to be straining under the weight of a monster barbell.

Most of the research into training during pregnancy has centred around aerobic activity rather than anaerobic, so there's little evidence of what works best for pregnant weight-lifters. But, given everything we know about the need to limit overheating, joint laxity and heart rate, I'd recommend shorter sets with lower intensity and weight. So, if you're an experienced weight-lifter, for example, you might continue to train at 65% of your 1RM ('one-rep max', i.e. the maximum you can lift just once). However, whereas pre-pregnancy you may have been doing 3 x 10 reps, you might adjust this now to 5 x 6 reps, or 6 x 5 sets. The idea is to achieve the same volume of training, but broken up in a way that's more compatible with your changing physiological needs.

After the first trimester, you'll need to replace bench press with incline bench press to avoid having to lie flat (best avoided after 20 weeks, as it can sometimes impede the blood flow through the body's biggest vein, the vena cava). Most importantly, watch your breathing technique: never hold your breath while you're lifting weights at any stage in your exercise programme.

As time goes on, you might want to substitute resistance machines for free weights, which don't challenge your balance to quite the same extent. It's also a good idea to consider a sacroiliac support belt: this helps maintain pelvic stability and alignment while you exercise. I used one for running and weight training from about five months into my pregnancy, and for a few months after the birth, too.

As always, listen to your body: keep a watchful eye on how you're feeling as you work out, and raise any concerns with your doctor.

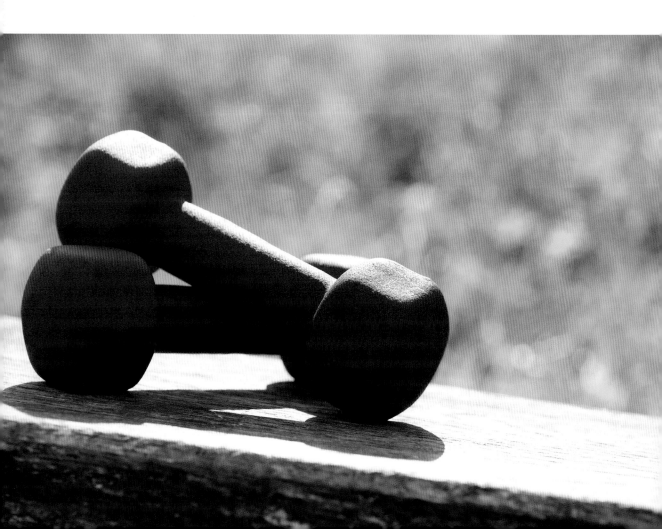

INTENSITY AND EFFORT

We used to hear a lot on the subject of the intensity at which women should train during pregnancy. In the recent past, medical personnel would advise that the maternal heart rate shouldn't go above 140 beats per minute (bpm). This was prompted by the fear that high core temperatures brought on by exercise would endanger the baby. But research has shown this not to be so much of a concern, because the natural restrictions that come with pregnancy usually serve as enough of a physical restraint! In other words, as your pregnancy runs its course, you'll find that your body will naturally dictate how much you can do.

The body is expert at prioritising its energy needs and will simply take everything it requires for the baby, as well as your own needs. Anything left in the tank is extra, so on days when its level is lower than usual, you'll feel slower, more tired and, therefore, naturally inclined to do a bit less. Don't stress about it; just accept the way you feel on these days as a signal to take it a little easier and help your body to get back on top of things. Of course, how comfortable you feel will vary according to how you are carrying, as well as the size of your bump. If you start feeling very uncomfortable, change your mode of exercise. If you were previously running, switch to power-walking; walk up hills rather than run them to avoid pushing your heart rate up; and run on softer surfaces to minimise the impact on your joints and bladder. However, remember that your ankle ligaments are more lax, too, so watch your footing and stick to a good, well-cushioned and supportive running shoe.

It's a good idea to wear a heart rate monitor whenever you're exercising and to know your upper limit (around 80% of your maximum number of beats per minute). Set the buzzer and don't go above this – if you reach it, slow down or walk until it drops.

What's absolutely certain is that this is definitely not the time to try to beat the clock. From four to five months into your pregnancy, decrease the intensity and volume of your training programme; run at a sedate pace and, if you feel puffed or tired, just walk. Don't on any account ignore warning signs and force yourself to keep going. And make very sure that you stay extra hydrated. Be careful, too, when you're stretching: there's a hormone at work called relaxin, which softens the ligaments and tendons in preparation for the birth. This can lull you into a sense of false confidence as regards your flexibility, and you may think you can stretch further than your limits. Err on the side of caution.

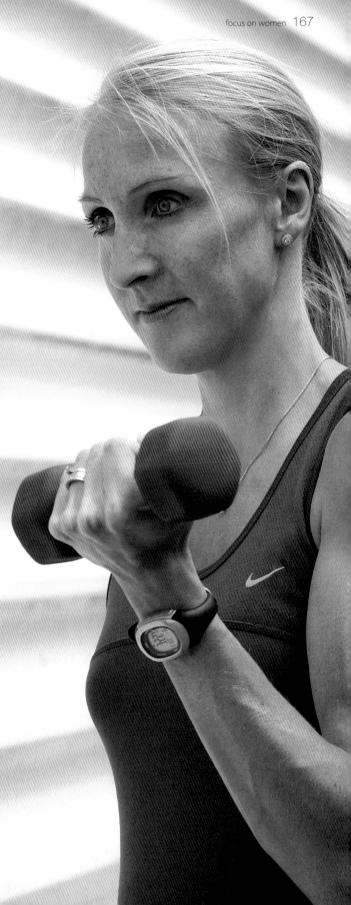

PELVIC FLOOR EXERCISES

If you've been lax about exercising your pelvic floor muscles, start without delay. (These are also called Kegel exercises, after Dr Arnold Kegel who invented them.) Your pelvic floor muscles (PFM) take extra strain and are weakened by having a baby pressing down on your bladder. But, like any other, they can be strengthened. Several muscles make up the PFM; collectively they act like a sling, supporting the uterus, bladder, intestines and the urinary and anal sphincters. From this description, it's easy to see why they play such a crucial role in preventing urinary leakage (sometimes referred to as 'stress incontinence').

The significance of weak pelvic floor muscles for runners – especially after you've had a baby – is that the jarring action of running can make you uncomfortably aware of small urinary leaks. Work on tightening them. You can practice these exercises anywhere and without anyone knowing you're doing them – you just have to remember to actually do them! Believe it or not, you can even concentrate on working them during your runs and while you are exercising.

First, though, you need to know where they are. Think of the muscles you squeeze when you're dying to go the loo – these are your pelvic floor muscles. To strengthen them, that's exactly what you do: squeeze them (you'll feel as though you're pulling them up higher into your body) and hold for five seconds before slowly releasing them. Don't tighten the abdominal muscles or the thigh muscles at the same time – you need to isolate the PFM and work them on their own. Start out doing about 25 reps per day, building to around 200. Seize any opportunity you find: standing at the sink, driving, on the bus, sitting or standing – there are plenty of moments during even the busiest schedule if you consciously look for them. In eight weeks you'll notice a difference.

'A sacro-ilioac support belt can double as a bump support when you get bigger'

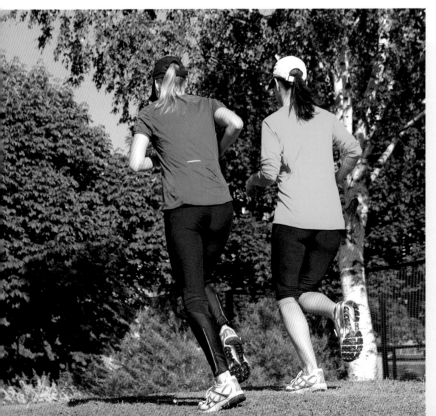

reminders...

Run with a friend who can keep an eye on how you're doing, and observe all the obvious safety measures – high visibility clothing; well-lit, frequented routes; with your iPod or MP3 player volume low so that you can hear what's going on around you. If you're alone, take a well-charged mobile with you at all times.

If you have any discomfort or concerns of any sort, stop and immediately see a doctor. My advice is to talk to your doctor as soon as you know you're pregnant and acquaint them with your training schedule. Keep them advised of any changes you make to your programme as you go along and, obviously, any changes in the way you feel.

EATING AND DRINKING FOR TWO?

When you're pregnant you need to consume about 300kcals more than usual per day to fuel your baby's development. As we know, baby comes first in the race for food. If you don't eat properly, it siphons off whatever it needs from your intake of food, leaving you feeling like a desiccated husk! If it fails to get enough nutrients from your diet, it will even leach calcium from your bones to make sure that it has enough, increasing your odds of osteoporosis later in life. So, pay attention to the nutritional content of what you eat. It's a good idea to increase your calcium and iron intake, or take them as supplements alongside your pre-natal vitamins. Be sure to get a good high intake of essential fatty acids; omega-3 in particular is very good for baby's brain and neural development. (Look back at Chapter 9, Eat to win, for food sources, and talk to a nutritionist before you start on a course of supplements.)

Once you get beyond the first trimester and any symptoms of nausea that you may have been experiencing fade away, this won't be difficult. I loved canned salmon with the bones and skin (great source of calcium and essential fats) mixed with avocado on baked potato or sandwiches for lunch. During those first three months, eat little and often as best you can. When you're training, a carbohydrate drink can sometimes help, although be careful that the sports drinks you consume have no added ingredients that you should avoid, such as caffeine. There might be a tussle between a craving for chocolate muffins and the nagging feeling that you should really be eating more nutritiously, but don't worry about it too much – just do what you can; the odd treat in moderation is good for us all. By the second trimester, the hormone changes will most likely have settled down and you'll feel quite differently about food. Having said that, though, you might start experiencing a touch of heartburn as baby takes up more and more space. As this happens, switch to grazing, i.e. eating little and often.

Keep your hydration levels up and don't allow your body to overheat. During pregnancy, your core temperature is higher due to the fact that your baby dissipates its heat via your body, which absorbs it. If you get too hot, baby's temperature also rises, which is potentially dangerous. Don't run in hot weather – wait for the cool of evening or run in the early morning; start well hydrated and, if necessary, take water with you.

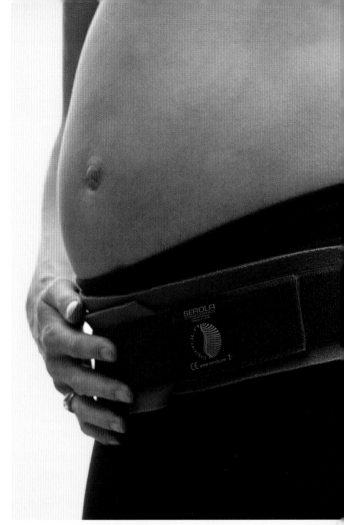

support clothing

As you expand, you'll be thinking about how to accommodate and support your bump when you're out running. Look for exercise clothing with a bit more give in the cut and a slightly more generous seam allowance to accommodate your growing tummy, but also for extra support and thickness around it. Shorts, running pants or leotards with extra-thick support around and under the bump are a godsend, although they are difficult to find. A sacroiliac support belt can also double as a bump support when you get bigger.

One very important requirement is a sports bra that offers very good support. If you've managed up until now with wearing just running tops with built-in bras or crop-tops, you'll find that at this stage you'll need more structure along the lines of the Shock Absorber range. Investing in the right bra is very important, not only throughout your pregnancy, but also for as long as you intend to breastfeed.

post-pregnancy

At this point, how much exercise you do will depend on how you feel and the type of birth you've had. Thanks to 'Nature's Prozac' (the near-miraculous effect of endorphins on our brain chemistry) there's no better antidote to baby blues than exercise.

Obviously, surgical procedures such as a caesarian will entail a longer recovery, whereas a vaginal birth with no complications will get you back to normal much faster. However, bear in mind that if you had an episiotomy, there will be stitches that need time to heal.

However, the one type of exercise you can start straight after the birth is Kegel exercises for your pelvic floor muscles (see page 168). In addition to these, as soon as you've fully healed and been cleared for action, you can also begin cautiously doing abdominal exercises. As for getting back to training, remember that it takes around six weeks for your body to return to its pre-pregnancy state.

After the birth of my daughter, I started with walking but progressed to easy running after just 12 days. I now know that was too soon; I still had internal swelling and trauma from the birth and, as I built up my training, my ligaments were not yet able to work properly and I ended up with a sacral stress fracture. Warning signs were achiness and pain in my lower back and lax bowel muscles during runs. Second time around, I know to give my body as long as it needs to recover and to listen carefully to how it responds once I do start running again. As a general rule of thumb, wait at least six weeks before you return to running after pregnancy. Start with regaining your core and posture with gentle conditioning and low impact work such as swimming, and perhaps consider a post-natal class to ease yourself back into it. A word of warning: be wary of too much elliptical training (the machine otherwise known as the cross-trainer), as this can put as much stress on the sacral area as running does.

One fun way to return to cardiovascular activity can be to join a group of other mums at a mum-and-buggy class. But remember, running while pushing a buggy isn't easy and uses your muscles differently from regular running, so be careful and build up very gradually. Done correctly, exercises that include pushing a buggy with baby in front of you are a terrific upper-body workout as well as a good reintroduction to aerobic exercise. Follow the manufacturer's advice as regards the age your baby should be before (s)he goes out in a jogger, as this can differ from brand to brand. Some recommend waiting until baby is at least 16 weeks old, as the vibration/movement can sometimes be harmful to small babies. Check the availability of these groups online, or get in touch with your local authority to see what's available.

After a surgical procedure such as a caesarian, you need to apply common sense: restraint and gradual build-up are the key words. Always get the go-ahead from your doctor or midwife before you start, and discuss with them how quickly you can train yourself back to full fitness again.

BREAST-FEEDING

Another big consideration, if you are breastfeeding, is milk supply. To feed successfully, you need to keep a bit more than your racing weight on board and eat around 500kcals more each day than the average daily requirements of 2,000kcals or so. You'll also need to drink extra fluid and make sure that the nutritional quality of your diet is sufficient to maintain good milk levels. It's a good idea to take a very good calcium supplement throughout this time. Despite rumours to the contrary, research tells us that exercising when you're breastfeeding makes no difference to how your milk tastes! Reports of lactic acid after hard training upsetting baby's taste buds are nonsense (though too much cabbage, spices or champagne might). I found it more comfortable to express or feed before runs – this also ensures that baby's next snack is there if you're late back. I also found that the bottle I expressed in the morning was creamier and richer, and giving my daughter this bottle before bed may have helped to get her to sleep through more quickly. It also stopped me stressing, as I often found my milk supply was weaker at the end of the day after training, because I was more tired. The other great benefit of breastfeeding is that it makes a difference to how quickly you get back to your pre-pregnancy weight and how quickly your uterus shrinks back to normal.

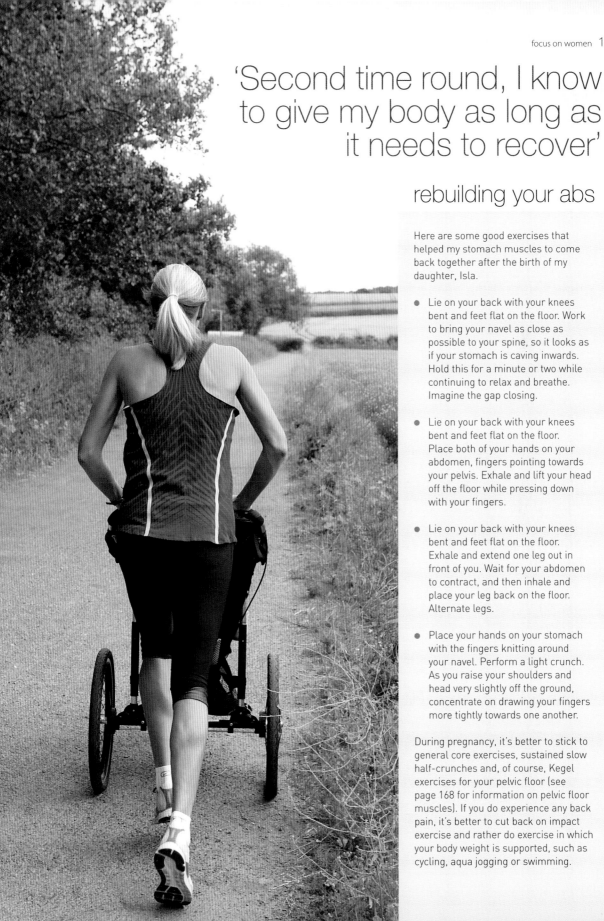

'Second time round, I know to give my body as long as it needs to recover'

rebuilding your abs

Here are some good exercises that helped my stomach muscles to come back together after the birth of my daughter, Isla.

- Lie on your back with your knees bent and feet flat on the floor. Work to bring your navel as close as possible to your spine, so it looks as if your stomach is caving inwards. Hold this for a minute or two while continuing to relax and breathe. Imagine the gap closing.

- Lie on your back with your knees bent and feet flat on the floor. Place both of your hands on your abdomen, fingers pointing towards your pelvis. Exhale and lift your head off the floor while pressing down with your fingers.

- Lie on your back with your knees bent and feet flat on the floor. Exhale and extend one leg out in front of you. Wait for your abdomen to contract, and then inhale and place your leg back on the floor. Alternate legs.

- Place your hands on your stomach with the fingers knitting around your navel. Perform a light crunch. As you raise your shoulders and head very slightly off the ground, concentrate on drawing your fingers more tightly towards one another.

During pregnancy, it's better to stick to general core exercises, sustained slow half-crunches and, of course, Kegel exercises for your pelvic floor (see page 168 for information on pelvic floor muscles). If you do experience any back pain, it's better to cut back on impact exercise and rather do exercise in which your body weight is supported, such as cycling, aqua jogging or swimming.

menopause

Exercise is believed to mitigate the symptoms that we associate with menopause. It's not only the uplifting effect on your mood caused by those much-mentioned endorphins, either – there are a few more good reasons for continuing to train once menopause has started.

Fighting abdominal fat

Fat – abdominal fat in particular – has a tendency to creep up on us at this point in our lives. But it needn't do, providing you keep on exercising. And for fat-burning purposes, there's little to beat running.

Prevention/slowing down of osteoporosis

During menopause, oestrogen levels drop dramatically. Oestrogen plays a key role in maintaining the health of our bones, keeping osteoclasts (which clear away old bone) in check and allowing osteoblasts (which create new bone) to build and strengthen our skeleton. When there isn't enough oestrogen to do this, bone density declines and the bones become weak and brittle. Unless you work to stop this, you can lose 2–7% of your bone mass every year. But you can take measures to ensure that you're not accelerating bone loss with a poor diet:

1 Build bone density right from the start

Young girls who run, plus their mothers, take note! Start building up bone density right from childhood and work at keeping it up throughout the teenage years and into the twenties. On average, we reach peak bone mass by our mid-twenties, after which our bone density slowly declines. When menopause hits, the decline accelerates. Make sure your youngsters get the right quantity and quality of food and plenty of impact and weight-bearing exercise (but not to the point where it delays the onset of menstruation). This will go a long way to starting young women off with the maximum bone mass, so that they minimise their chances of dipping below the level at which osteoporosis becomes a possibility.

2 Monitor your periods

Firstly, ensure that you're still having periods. This means checking that your energy intake (i.e. calories) is as good as it can be, and that you allow sufficient time to recover from training.

3 Audit your diet

We need about 1,200–1,500mg of calcium and 1,000iu of vitamin D per day, but the average Western diet contains as little as half that. So, the first thing to do is make sure that we're getting plenty of calcium, vitamin D, vitamin K, magnesium, manganese, boron and zinc. Seek advice from a nutritionist as to which is the best mineral supplement to help combat bone thinning. There are plenty out there, but you want to know which ones provide all the minerals, not just the major ones (calcium and vitamin D). Then review your diet and include foods that help supply the minerals you need.

4 Train with weights

Regular strength training using dumbbells, barbells, fixed-resistance machines, resistance bands or your own body weight has a marked effect on improving bone density. The key word here is 'regular' – three times a week is ideal. When you're lifting weights it's the action of muscles pulling against bones that seems to stimulate the building of bone, as well as helping maintain calcium levels in the bones that are handling the load. Bear in mind that weight-bearing exercise means activities that involve carrying at least your own body weight – cycling and swimming don't count, as you are supported on the bike and in the water. However, running, brisk walking and exercising on an elliptical machine (a.k.a. cross-trainer) do count, plus, of course, lifting weights.

Finally, the only accurate way to determine your bone density is via a bone scan. If your results reveal reduced bone density, remember that there are different levels of osteoporosis. Check that your training programme involves a level of impact that's appropriate to your individual condition. You'll also need to have repeat scans to assess the rate of decline. Talk to a sports physiologist about your exercise routine and keep a close watch on how you feel.

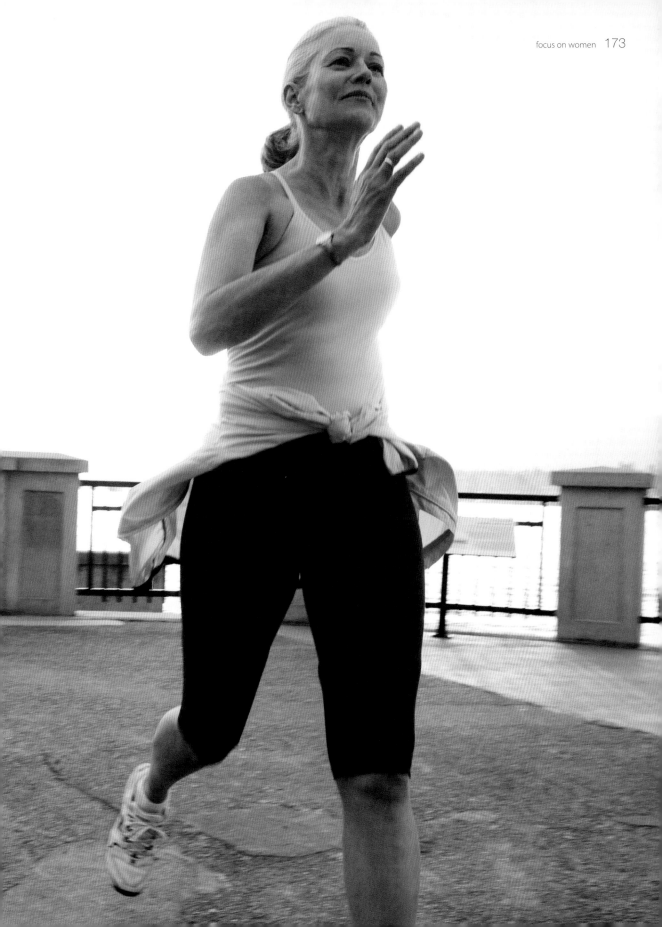

index

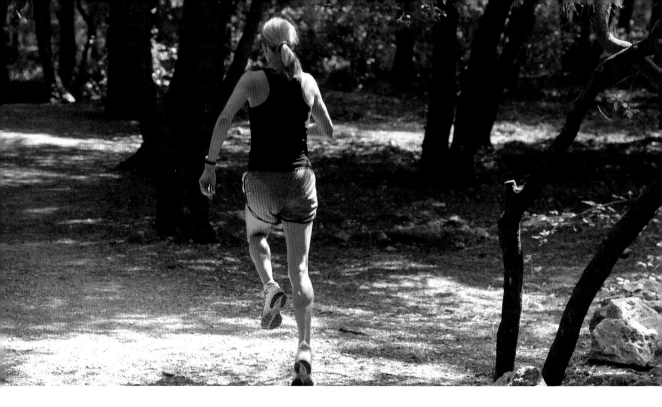

acknowledgments

My coach, Alex Stanton, who has guided me from the age of 11, has passed on so much of what I know. What sticks with me more than anything else is his conviction that in athletics you are never done with learning – and we often learn more from defeats and tough times than from victories. But we cannot know it all. Alex and his wife Rosemary were never afraid to ask for advice. He loved to sit down with great coaches such as Harry Wilson and pick their brains. No wonder Alex's philosophy is so important to me. In short, it goes like this: running should be fun; always be honest with yourself; be in tune with your body; never be afraid to listen to your gut instincts. Before a big race, he'd invariably reinforce these injunctions by saying: 'You're in great shape, you're the one out there racing, and you have the racing brain. Go and enjoy yourself!'

Throughout my career, many people have given me invaluable advice, which I have tried to pass on in this book. The list is long and humbling: I've had the loving support of my family, and Alex and Rosemary; top-class input from weights coach Max Jones; and the weight-training expertise at the Michael Johnson Performance Center in Texas. Then there's the injury prevention and rehab I've received, not to mention the sports anatomy knowledge gained through working with great physiotherapists and sports medical specialists such as Mark Buckingham, Vaughan Cooper, Yannick Guillaumet, Gerard Hartman, Andy Jones, Al Kupczak, Dana Paine, Michel Riff, Dr Amol Saxena, Rone Thompson, Justin Whittaker and Dr Hans-Wilhelm Müller-Wohlfahrt.

I don't know how to put into words the wisdom I've picked up over the years from getting the chance to sit, chat with and learn from world-class athletes such as Steve Cram, Seb Coe, Steve Ovett, Alberto Salazar, Ingrid Kristiansen, Grete Waitz, Joanie Benoit Samuelson, Liz McColgan and many more. The running world can be likened to one big family of kindred spirits who share a common love. My goal and, I'm sure, that of many other athletes is to pass on this passion to others, especially children, so that they, too, can grow and flourish through sport and running.

A sincere note of appreciation to Nike for their huge support; for valuing my feedback; for letting me contribute to footwear, apparel and eyewear design; and for sharing research findings.

In pregnancy and motherhood, I have to thank my daughter Isla, son Raphael, husband Gary, parents and parents-in-law for always being there for me. Also, Dr Michael Dooley for his gynaecological advice on safe training in pregnancy, and to Drs Fayad and Demetrescu and the Centre Hospitalier Princesse Grace in Monaco for their expert support through pregnancies, deliveries and recoveries.

Finally a big, big thank-you to photographic team Ruth Jenkinson and Carly Churchill, creative director Nigel Wright, writer and editor Hilary Ivory and publishers Simon & Schuster for helping me produce this book and get it out to you. I really hope you enjoy it and find it useful.